The Effects of Various Diseases on the Development of Atherosclerosis

The Effects of Various Diseases on the Development of Atherosclerosis

Anatoliĭ M. Vikhert
and Valentin S. Zhdanov

English Language Edition Edited by
James E. Muller

Pergamon Press
New York Oxford Toronto Sydney Frankfurt Paris

Pergamon Press Offices:

U.S.A. Pergamon Press Inc., Maxwell House, Fairview Park, Elmsford, New York 10523, U.S.A.

U.K. Pergamon Press Ltd., Headington Hill Hall, Oxford OX3 OBW, England

CANADA Pergamon of Canada, Ltd., Suite 104, 150 Consumers Road, Willowdale, Ontario M2J 1P9, Canada

AUSTRALIA Pergamon Press (Aust.) Pty. Ltd., P.O. Box 544, Potts Point, NSW 2011, Australia

FRANCE Pergamon Press SARL, 24 rue des Ecoles, 75240 Paris, Cedex 05, France

FEDERAL REPUBLIC OF GERMANY Pergamon Press GmbH, Hammerweg 6, Postfach 1305, 6242 Kronberg/Taunus, Federal Republic of Germany

Translated from the Russian *Ateroskleroz pri razlichnykh zabolevaniiakh*. Moscow, Meditsina, 1976.
Translated and printed under the Special Foreign Currency Program of the National Library of Medicine, National Institutes of Health, Public Health Service, U.S. Department of Health and Human Services, pursuant to an agreement with the National Science Foundation, Washington, D.C., by Amerind Publishing Co., Pvt. Ltd., New Delhi

Library of Congress Cataloging in Publication Data

Vikhert, Anatolii Mikhailovich.
The effects of various diseases on the development of atherosclerosis.

Translation of Ateroskleroz pri razlichnykh zabolevaniiakh.
Bibliography: 19 p.
Includes index.
1. Atherosclerosis. 2. Diseases—Complications and sequelae. 3. Autopsy.
I. Zhdanov, Valentin S., joint author. II. Muller, James E. III. Title. [DNLM:
1. Arteriosclerosis—Complications. WG550 V694a]
RC692.V5413 1980 616.1′36071 80-13069
ISBN 0-08-025555-8

Printed in India at Eastend Printers, Calcutta

Preface to the English Edition

The problems of cardiovascular diseases are currently receiving worldwide attention. They are major health problems, shared to a greater or lesser degree by all nations, both industrialized and developing.

International cooperation in sharing of data is important in gaining new insights about the relative contributions of various factors in the development and prevention of these diseases. More than ever before medical science is international in scope and character. Through international cooperation, the talents, insights, and experience of many nations is being brought to bear on these worldwide disease problems. The book on "Atherosclerosis in Various Diseases" is a timely and comprehensive contribution of Soviet research to these international efforts. It presents the problem of atherosclerosis from a novel perspective. The authors examine the impact that various other diseases have on the pathogenesis and development of atherosclerosis, thereby providing new clues to these problems. These studies also pose new questions requiring further scientific investigation.

This book is the second major translation undertaken in the spirit of the US-USSR collaboration in cardiovascular diseases. Professor Anatolii Mikhailovich Vikhert is the Soviet coordinator for one of the collaborative research areas within the US-USSR joint program. The cardiovascular program was initiated in 1972 under a five-year Agreement between the Government of the United States and the Government of the Union of Soviet Socialist Republics in the field of Medical Science and Public Health. This agreement represented the culmination of a long series of contacts and exchanges between medical scientists and physicians in the two countries. The agreement was renewed in 1977 for a second term of five years.

Funds for the translation and publication of this book were provided through the International Programs Division of the National Library of Medicine, NIH. Funds for editing of the English language translation, which was carried out by Dr. James E. Muller, were provided by the National Heart, Lung, and Blood Institute, NIH.

Ruth Johnsson Hegyeli, M.D.
Assistant Director for International Programs
National Heart, Lung, and Blood Institute

Introduction to the English Edition

In addition to their positions as the nuclear superpowers of the world, the United States and the Soviet Union share the problem of an extremely high prevalence of atherosclerosis. This book describes original research conducted in the Soviet Union which should be of interest to investigators throughout the world who are concerned with the problem of atherosclerosis.

The book describes the results of a standardized autopsy study of atherosclerosis in 6,417 patients and 2,625 essentially healthy individuals who suffered an accidental death. Not only do the authors have a large enough sample size to draw many conclusions, but they also have been extremely careful to select the proper groups for comparison and to control for the effects of sex and age on the atherosclerotic process.

The major focus of the study is on the characteristics of atherosclerosis in combination with other diseases (diabetes mellitus, malignant neoplasms, cirrhosis of the liver, rheumatic heart disease, chronic lung disease, pulmonary tuberculosis, thyrotoxicosis, and hypertension). With these comparisons certain intriguing relationships emerge, such as the accelerated atherosclerosis in the thoracic aorta of patients with chronic lung disease and the reduced calcification of plaques in patients with renal hypertension.

A feature of the book of special value to English-speaking investigators is the extensive bibliography which provides an opening to previously unrecognized Soviet research.

It is hoped that the translation of this book into English will assist in bringing data and insights from the Soviet Union to the worldwide struggle against this far too prevalent disease.

James E. Muller, M.D.

Foreword

In the second half of the twentieth century atherosclerotic lesions of the arteries have become a most important health problem. The incidence of atherosclerosis has been rising continuously all over the world, not only in certain countries, but on all the continents, so that the problem assumes a global character. Atherosclerosis is the single leading cause of death; its complications are the cause of death in 30 to 40% of the male population. Because of its wide prevalence, the coexistence of atherosclerosis with other diseases is the rule rather than the exception. However, little is known of the effect of various diseases on the origin, formation and course of atherosclerosis and the development of its various complications. At the same time, the importance and urgency of this problem for clinical and theoretical cardiology cannot be denied.

The available works on this problem are contradictory, not comparable and small in number. So it is impossible to draw any definite conclusions from existing data. Confusion results from the absence of a uniform method of study of the materials at the disposal of different authors and the difficulty of forming comparable groups. A special center for the study of the epidemiology and pathology of atherosclerosis has been organized in the Soviet Union; this center has collected and summarized unique data.

This monograph contains the first detailed information on the effect of various diseases on the course of atherosclerosis in general and coronary atherosclerosis in particular. The data are expressed with a completely objective quantitative method. Extensive use of mathematics has been made to provide quantitative expression of the findings. It may be noted that in different spheres of medicine mathematical methods are continually gaining importance. When pathological processes can be expressed numerically they become tangible: objective expression of this can be seen in this book.

The authors have not presented data concerning the etiology and pathogenesis of atherosclerosis since this does not fall within the scope of this work. We know or we think that the morphological, biochemical and clinical manifestations of atherosclerosis are already known, but it should be admitted that at present our knowledge of the pathogenesis of atherosclerosis has virtually reached a deadlock. To understand the pathogenesis of this disease new methods and new approaches are necessary; it will be necessary to solve the pathogenesis of atherosclerosis on a subcellular or molecular level, on the level of vascular and cellular membranes, as is the modern trend of research. This research is already in progress and the authors of this monograph are participating in it.

Apart from the problems of pathogenesis, many other aspects of the development of atherosclerosis in man remain unclear. The research carried out by the authors elucidates some of them. A study showing the characteristics of the course of the atherosclerotic process depending on various diseases reveals the significance of a number of factors in atherogenesis. This presentation of the morphometric characteristics of atherosclerosis in patients with various diseases, taking into account their age, sex, and qualitative features of the atherosclerotic process, is completely original.

The book is recommended for a wide group of physicians of various specialties, including internists, cardiologists, pathologists, and practically all those interested in studying this problem. It will undoubtedly be received with interest by the medical community.

Academician E. I. Chazov
USSR Academy of Medical Sciences

Contents

Introduction

Atherosclerosis is one of the most important problems in modern medicine. The death rate and cause of death of many patients over 50 years old are connected with various manifestations of atherosclerosis. In the last 15 to 20 years a steady growth of diseases connected with atherosclerosis has also been noted in younger individuals; this is known as atherosclerosis of youth. Atherosclerosis has an intimate relationship with ischemic heart disease, hypertension, and cerebrovascular disease.

Although research has been conducted for many years, numerous problems concerning the etiology and pathogenesis of atherosclerosis have yet to be solved. This radically affects the prophylaxis and treatment of these diseases. The study of the atherosclerotic process and its qualitative and quantitative features in subjects with various diseases is of great importance for identification of the factors and conditions that promote or, on the other hand, retard the development of this process.

The relationship of atherosclerosis to other diseases also has practical significance. With the advent of modern treatment of several diseases (diabetes mellitus, pulmonary tuberculosis, chronic pneumonia, rheumatic heart disease) the length of life has been considerably increased, which to a great extent explains the rise in atherosclerosis in association with other diseases that has been noted in recent times.

Morphological studies of atherosclerosis have been the most consistent, although there are many contradictory reports of the characteristics of atherosclerosis, based on the study of autopsy materials. These discrepancies result primarily from the subjective evaluation of atherosclerosis at the time of autopsy. This results partly from the absence of a generally accepted method for determining the stages and the degree of atherosclerosis and from the heterogeneity of the groups studied. Since there are considerable individual variations in the manifestation of atherosclerosis, well-founded and valid conclusions characterizing atherosclerosis can be obtained only by studying a sufficiently large number of observations with adequate homogeneity of the groups studied.

This application of objective methods to the quantitative study of atherosclerosis in specific, strictly localized parts of the arterial systems, using unified terminology and techniques for preparing the specimens, is a new advance in the study of atherosclerosis in autopsy materials (Avtandilov, 1960; Buvailo, 1960; Smolenskii, 1960; Vikhert *et al.*, 1965; Tejada *et al.*, 1958; Kagan and Uemura, 1962). The quantitative study of the atherosclerotic process can be used to express the law of its development in mathematical and statistical terms. This is particularly important, since many phenomena in biology and medicine follow statistical rules. This is noticeable only when we study them in totality, since these rules are not applicable to an isolated individual belonging to this totality (Plokhinskii, 1961; Bessmertnyi, 1967; Bailey, 1962).

As a rule study of the problems of the pathogenesis and epidemiology of atherosclerosis involves conducting a comparative study of atherosclerotic changes in various groups of people or animals. This requires not only a uniform classification of the changes, but also a comprehensive idea of the different terms of the same type of processes. In the absence of an agreement on classification and terminology it is impossible to compare the results obtained in different investigations. Unfortunately there are many classifications of atherosclerotic changes (Anichkov, 1947; Davydovskii, 1958; Tejada *et al.*, 1958; Abrikosov and Strusov, 1961; Moses, 1963; Mitchell and Schwartz, 1965), differing both in the choice of terminology and in choice of types of change.

On the initiative of the World Health Organization (WHO) a study group of pathologists from different countries worked out methodological principles for the conduct of comparative quantitative examination of atherosclerosis in autopsy materials. These principles are used in the present work. Since different pathologists define the degree of atherosclerosis differently even in the same case, it was decided to preserve the vessels for the whole period of examination in plastic bags at the time of autopsy. This allows us to study the atherosclerosis in the vessels in which we are interested under standard conditions and to repeat the examination in the same vessels in order to check the degree of reproducibility of the results of evaluation of atherosclerosis.

A quantitative study of the qualitative features of the atherosclerotic process—lipidosis, fibrous plaques, complicated lesions, and calcification—in some parts of a vascular system reveals information about the development of atherosclerosis in certain conditions and diseases. The WHO study group of pathologists has recommended using the following parts of the vascular system to solve the problems of the epidemiology and pathology of atherosclerosis: descending thoracic aorta, abdominal aorta, right coronary artery, circumflex and descending branches of the left coronary artery (WHO Standard Working Protocol, Moscow, 1962).

In 1962 a special center for study of the epidemiology and pathology of atherosclerosis was established in the USSR in the department of Pathology of the Institute of Therapy, Academy of Medical Sciences. This center participated in a program in collaboration with WHO. In conformity with this program, in this investigation we have presented the results of the study of the above parts of vessels with the following boundaries:

Descending thoracic aorta—from a horizontal line drawn through the first two intercostal arteries to a horizontal line drawn through the upper edge of the orifice of the celiac artery.

Abdominal aorta—from a horizontal line drawn through the upper edge of the orifice of the celiac artery to a horizontal line drawn through the bifurcation of the aorta.

Right coronary artery—from the orifice (inclusive) to the midpoint of the posterior descending branch of this artery (excluding all the lateral branches).

Left circumflex coronary artery—from the origin, excluding the auxiliary branches, to the farthest traceable point.

Left anterior descending coronary artery—from the orifice (inclusive) to the apex of the left ventricle (excluding the lateral branches).

When describing the changes in the above vessels we used the pathological terms as defined by the WHO study group of pathologists.

Atherosclerosis—a variable combination of changes in the intima of arteries, characterized by focal accumulation of lipids, complex carbohydrates, blood and its products with the development of a fibrous tissue and deposit of calcium salts and associated with media changes.

Fatty streaks—any intimal lesion that is distinctly stained with Sudan VI and does not show any other changes in the other layers of a vessel wall.

Fibrous plaques—firm, glistening (occasionally translucent), white or pale gray colored thickening of intima. These plaques may not be stained or may be stained partially or completely with Sudan. If a lesion presents any hemorrhage, thrombosis, erosion or calcification, then such changes are classified in the respective categories, but not as fibrous plaques.

Complicated lesions—areas of intima with hemorrhages, erosions and thrombosis, with or without the deposit of calcium salts.

Calcification—areas where deposits of calcium salts are detectable visually or by palpation, in the absence of hemorrhages, erosions, or thrombosis.

Moreover, in this work the term *raised lesions* includes fibrous plaques, complicated lesions, and calcification.

The quantitative evaluation of atherosclerotic changes utilized in the present study consisted in determining the area of the intimal surface of a vessel occupied by fatty streaks, fibrous plaques, complicated lesions, or calcification, and similarly the percentage of the total areas of these changes in relation to the intimal surface of a vessel. To calculate the areas showing the above changes we utilized the visual-planimetric method of evaluation (Vikhert *et al.*, 1966), which essentially consists of the following: A grid marked with a jotter pen is placed over the plastic bags where the aorta or coronary arteries are stored. Each division of this corresponds to a specific part of a vessel: 50%,

25%, 12%, 6%, 1%. Then with the help of this planimetric scale we visually determine the area occupied by the various types of atherosclerotic changes. The precision of determination of the areas of various types of change is about 1%. Based on visual study the presence or absence of narrowing of the lumen of the coronary arteries by 50% or more is also noted. About 20% of the specimens are studied a second time either by the same or by another pathologist under the same conditions. When carrying out the first or subsequent evaluations of the atherosclerotic changes in the vessels the pathologist has no knowledge of the cases from which the vessels were collected. To explain the peculiarities of the course of atherosclerosis in certain groups of people, not only the areas but also the prevalence of the atherosclerotic changes are determined. On the basis of the presence of various types of change the atherosclerotic process has been subdivided into the following stages: stage I—only fatty streaks in the vessels; stage II—fatty streaks and fibrous plaques; stage III—the changes characteristic of stage II plus complicated lesions; stage IV—the changes characteristic of stage III plus calcification; stage V—complicated lesions and calcification.

The results of the evaluations of atherosclerosis are entered on special cards (separately for aorta and coronary arteries) bearing the same serial number as that of the vessels in the plastic bag. Prof. A. M. Vikhert, Dr. V. S. Zhdanov, and Dr. E. E. Matova from Moscow; Dr. A. M. Lifshits from Yalta; Prof. R. Vanecek and Dr. Z. Zagorzh from Prague, Czechoslovakia; Prof. N. Sternby and Dr. S. Lunberg from Malmö, Sweden, participated in the evaluation of specimens collected from Tallin, Tartu, Ryazan, Yalta, and Kishinev. The results obtained by repeated examination and cross-checking of the vessels by the same and also by different pathologists indicate their reproducibility in the highest degree. Deviations between the first and second evaluation for the determination of an area of complicated lesions and calcification on an average were not higher than 1–1.5%. Deviations for lipidosis and fibrous plaques were 1.5–2% and 3–4%, respectively. The repeated examination of atherosclerosis in the same vessels by the visual-planimetric and planimetric methods indicates that both methods are suitable for reproducing the results of evaluation to the necessary degree of precision (Lifshits *et al.*, 1966).

For each observation the pathologist or specialist completed a special card containing the clinicomorphological information relating to the epidemiology and pathology of atherosclerosis. The following important information about the deceased, necessary for analysis of the data, had already been incorporated: date of death, autopsy number, name of the hospital, permanent residence (urban or rural), nature of death (expected or unexpected), clinical diagnosis, age, sex, thickness of the subcutaneous fat in the standard area, weight of the heart, presence or absence of hypertension, diabetes mellitus, syphilis, thrombosis of cerebral arteries, myocardial infarction, cardiosclerosis, nature of cerebral circulation, diseases of peripheral vessels, pathological diagnosis. As stated above, these data were not supplied to the pathologist at the time of evaluation of the vessels.

In this work we present the materials of a study on atherosclerotic changes in the aorta and coronary arteries in the following diseases: diabetes mellitus (403 cases), malignant tumors (1,803 cases), cirrhosis of the liver (203 cases), rheumatic heart disease (408 cases), chronic, nonspecific inflammatory diseases of the lungs (329 cases), chronic pulmonary tuberculosis (318 cases), thyrotoxicosis (63 cases), essential hypertension (1,682 cases) and renal hypertension (684 cases).

The data showing the atherosclerotic changes in the diseases studied are compared either with the manifestation in healthy individuals (2,625 cases), or in persons dying from various types of complications of atherosclerosis (837 cases). Obviously the above groups served in the present work as control groups. The materials presented in this book were received by the center for the study of epidemiology and pathology from Moscow, Ryazan, Tallin, Tartu, Kaunas, Kharkov, and Yalta. Some materials from Kishinev and Irkutsk collected in the period from 1963 through 1966 were also used. The present work analyzes the occurrence of atherosclerosis in a total of 7,049 necropsies.

During the statistical analysis of the data for quantitative evaluation of atherosclerosis we calculated the mean prevalence and extent of various types of atherosclerotic changes in 10-year age groups, separately for males and females. For the convenience of comparing the manifestation of atherosclerosis in various groups of people we also determined the age-standardized index and in some cases the atherosclerotic index, as suggested by Holman *et al.* (1958). The latter represents the sum of half of the total area showing calcification and complicated lesions and a fourth of the area of fibrous plaques (as a percentage of the intimal surface of the vessels studied).

The statistically significant differences between the indices were calculated with the help of the Student 't' test (differences were considered significant when $p \leqslant 0.05$). To demonstrate the difference between the groups in the manifestation of atherosclerosis we sometimes utilized nonparametric criteria, particularly criteria of signs (KS) and the paired criteria of Wilcoxon (Gubler and Genkin, 1973).

A comparison of the manifestation of atherosclerotic changes in persons with various diseases and its manifestation in healthy individuals and in people dying from atherosclerosis as the main cause of illness helped us to identify the characteristics of the development of atherosclerosis in various groups. We were able to analyze the rate of development of the process, and some of its qualitative differences. The latter are primarily expressed by changes in the quantitative relations between separate types of atherosclerotic changes. When analyzing the characteristics of the course of atherosclerosis in persons dying from various diseases we considered the information available in the literature dealing with clinical and biochemical features of these diseases.

1

Dynamics of the Development of Atherosclerotic Changes in the Aorta and Coronary Arteries

Characterization of atherosclerosis in various groups of people is important for an explanation of the role of various factors in the development of atherosclerotic changes. Pathologists have an opportunity to study atherosclerosis in people dying from non-atherosclerotic diseases. The atherosclerotic changes in the vessels in the presence of certain diseases are usually compared with the heterogeneous atherosclerosis in all other types of death. Hence comparative investigations of atherosclerosis and the effect of various diseases on its course have often proved contradictory. For comparative studies the group of essentially healthy individuals (EHI) should be as homogeneous as possible. The atherosclerotic changes in such a group of individuals are the most representative of the natural development of atherosclerosis in a particular city or geographical area. This suggests that the EHI group is adequate as a control group and therefore useful for studying the characteristics of the development of atherosclerosis in various pathological conditions. In addition, the data on the characteristics of atherosclerosis in this group may be used to conduct comparative epidemiological studies of atherosclerosis in different cities.

In the group of essentially healthy individuals were included cases that satisfied the following requirements: (1) sudden death (mostly traumatic); (2) no changes in the internal organs indicating the presence of chronic diseases; (3) absence of post-infarction scars in the myocardium, obliteration or thrombosis of coronary arteries, or signs of an acute or old cerebrovascular accident on autopsy; (4) weight of heart not more than 400 g in males and not more than 350 g in females. (These weights, according to our findings, are the upper limit of the normal range in this group with average heart weights of 330 g in males and 290 g in females.)

Some data showing the nature of atherosclerosis in EHI are available in the literature (Anichkov, 1935; Roberts *et al.*, 1959; Grosse, 1960; Avtandilov, 1965, 1970; Sternby, 1968). These works were based on small studies, which used various classifications of the atherosclerotic changes. Various ways of expressing the process (e.g., analysis of the case history, measurement of the area of atherosclerotic changes in vessels stained and not stained with Sudan) were used for analyzing these materials. These differences affected the qualitative characteristics of the process in people belonging to this group.

In Table 1 we present data collected from various cities showing the average manifestation of atherosclerosis in the aorta and coronary arteries in EHI. The data were obtained by the Center for the Study of the Epidemiology and Pathology of Atherosclerosis, and the cases are shown distributed according to age and sex.

Table 1. Age and Sex Distribution of Essentially Healthy Individuals with Atherosclerosis

Age in years	10–19	20–29	30–39	40–49	50–59	60–69	70–79	Total
Male	97	505	585	328	248	142	76	1981
Female	30	109	125	115	120	86	59	644

For each age-sex group we calculated the mean statistical indices of an area showing the types of lesions and the prevalence of various stages of any atherosclerotic process. The earliest atherosclerotic changes are fatty streaks and fibrous plaques. Their localization in the vessels was to a certain extent dependent on the hemodynamic factors acting on the wall of a vessel (Anichkov, 1947; Davydovskii, 1958, 1967; Badmaeva, 1963; Doerr, 1963; Smolenskii, 1964; Glagov, 1965).

In both parts of the aorta the atherosclerotic changes appear early, and by the second or third decade of life they are found in 98–99% of cases. In the second decade of life fatty streaks in the aorta are found in more than 92% of cases and fibrous plaques in only 5–7% of cases. In third, fourth, and fifth decades of life the number of vessels with fibrous plaques increases and the number of vessels with only fatty streaks decreases (Table 2). By the fifth decade of life fibrous plaques in the thoracic aorta are found in almost half of all cases. In the abdominal aorta fibrous plaques appear early, and by the fifth decade of life more than 60% of EHIs have fibrous plaques in their abdominal aorta. Complicated lesions and calcification appear in isolated cases in the third decade of life. The number of such cases increases with age and by the seventh and eighth decades of life such changes are found in the aortas of most subjects.

Analysis of the prevalence of various stages of atherosclerosis in the aorta revealed that certain variations depend on sex: more severe stages of atherosclerosis were noticeable in both parts of the aorta of males in the fourth, fifth, sixth, and seventh decades of life compared to female cases. In the extreme age groups (second, third, and eighth decades of life) the variations in the prevalence of stages of aortic atherosclerosis between the sexes are not so high. Only in the eighth decade of life were complicated lesions often seen in females in the thoracic aorta (see Table 2).

Table 2. Prevalence: Stages of Atherosclerosis in Thoracic and Abdominal Aortas in Essentially Healthy Individuals

Age in years	Sex	Thoracic aorta			Abdominal aorta		
		Stage I*	Stage II	Stages III & IV	Stage I	Stage II	Stages III & IV
10–19	Male	92.0	8.0	—	92.7	7.3	—
	Female	92.3	7.7	—	85.9	11.3	—
20–29	Male	86.9	12.7	0.4	79.7	20.0	0.3
	Female	85.4	13.0	0.8	80.0	18.4	0.8
30–39	Male	69.2	29.6	0.9	43.9	53.6	2.5
	Female	79.6	19.5	0.9	60.2	38.9	0.9
40–49	Male	44.8	48.2	6.6	15.4	65.0	19.6
	Female	49.0	47.0	3.0	25.6	62.7	11.7
50–59	Male	17.2	63.8	19.0	7.3	46.4	46.5
	Female	15.4	65.0	12.6	9.4	56.2	35.4
60–69	Male	3.4	51.3	45.3	2.0	21.5	76.5
	Female	1.2	59.7	39.1	—	41.5	58.5
70–79	Male	1.4	40.3	58.3	1.4	14.1	84.5
	Female	—	26.4	73.6	—	20.7	79.3

* Atherosclerosis Stage I, only lipidosis in the vessels; Stage II, lipidosis in combination with fibrous plaques; Stages III and IV, vessels with complicated lesions and/or calcification. Figures are percent of cases in each group.

The development of atherosclerotic changes in coronary arteries has some peculiarities. By the second or third decade of life the aorta showed atherosclerotic changes in nearly all cases. However, coronary arteries without atherosclerotic changes were often seen in these decades, and in a small number of cases coronary arteries without any changes were noted up to the seventh decade of life (Table 3; Fig. 1). The atherosclerotic changes were seen most frequently in the left anterior descending (LAD) coronary artery and rarely in the right and circumflex coronary arteries. Fatty streaks were often noted as the only lesions; lipidosis was the main type of change in coronary arteries in the second, third, and fourth decades of life and even in the eighth decade of life lipidosis was the major change in 4% of males and 2% of females.

Table 3. Prevalence of EHI Cases Without Atherosclerotic Changes in the Right Coronary Artery and LAD Coronary Artery (Percentage of Number of Cases in Groups)

Vessels	Sex	10–19	20–29	30–39	40–49	50–59	60–69
Right coronary artery	Male	47.3*	31.1	15.9	5.0	1.7	2.1
	Female	60.8	36.2	29.9	13.4	10.7	1.2
LAD coronary artery	Male	28.2	13.4	3.2	2.0	0.4	0.7
	Female	40.0	17.2	8.5	5.0	1.1	1.2

* Percent of cases in each age group.

Fibrous plaques in coronary arteries are often found in the second decade of life, and by the fourth they are found in the LAD coronary artery in the majority of EHI. Coronary arteries with complicated lesions and calcification were seen in most cases only in subjects older than 70 years (Table 4; Fig. 1). Attention is drawn to the fact that the changes characterizing more severe stages of the atherosclerotic process, particularly fibrous plaques, complicated lesions, and calcification, are more often seen in the vessels of males than of females; only in subjects over 70 years does this difference disappear.

Table 4. Prevalence of Atherosclerosis in LAD Coronary Artery in EHI

Age in years	Stage I		Stage II		Stages III and IV	
	Male	Female	Male	Female	Male	Female
10–19	53.0*	51.1	18.8	8.9	—	—
20–29	38.2	52.5	48.1	30.3	0.3	—
30–39	25.6	35.8	68.5	55.7	2.7	—
40–49	11.3	27.0	75.8	64.0	10.9	4.0
50–59	6.9	18.7	65.5	59.5	27.2	20.9
60–69	2.1	8.7	52.5	54.3	44.7	35.8
70–79	4.3	2.0	37.7	36.0	58.0	62.0

* Percent of cases in each age-sex group. Stage I, lipidosis; Stage II, fibrous plaques; Stages III and IV, complicated lesions and/or calcification.

The total area of atherosclerotic changes increases with age in all vessels, but the changes are maximal in the abdominal aorta and the LAD coronary artery. They are minimal in the thoracic aorta and left circumflex coronary artery (Fig. 2). The differences between males and females in the total area

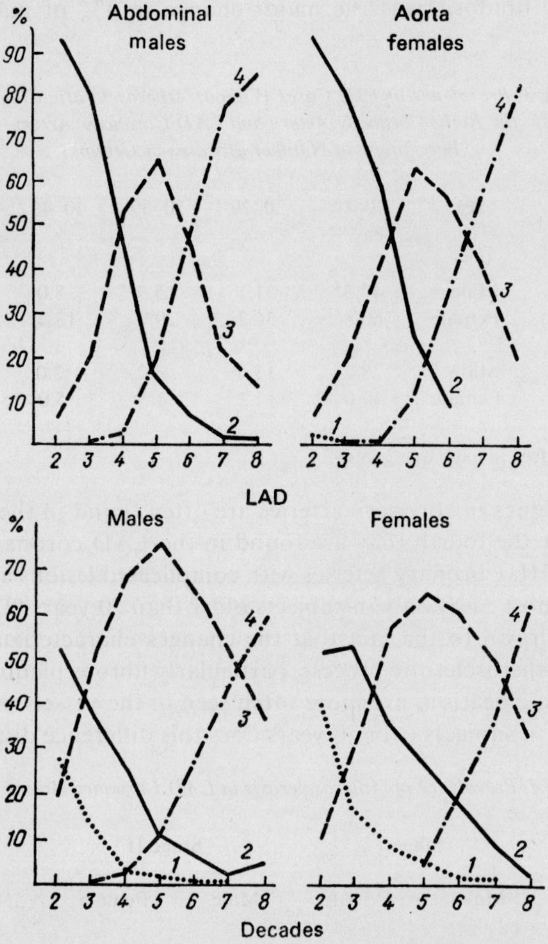

Figure 1. Prevalence of various stages of atherosclerosis in abdominal aorta and in the left anterior descending coronary artery in EHI.

The ordinate shows the prevalence of stages of atherosclerosis (percentage of observations). Curve *1*, vessels showing no change; *2*, vessels with lipidosis only; *3*, vessels with lipidosis and fibrous plaques; *4*, vessels with complicated lesions and/or calcification.

with atherosclerotic changes in the thoracic and abdominal aorta are not very high and statistically are not significant, but the total area with atherosclerotic changes was somewhat greater in the ages up to 70 years in males and above 70 years in females. In the coronary arteries of males the total area of atherosclerotic changes is usually greater, but here, too, differences are not always statistically significant.

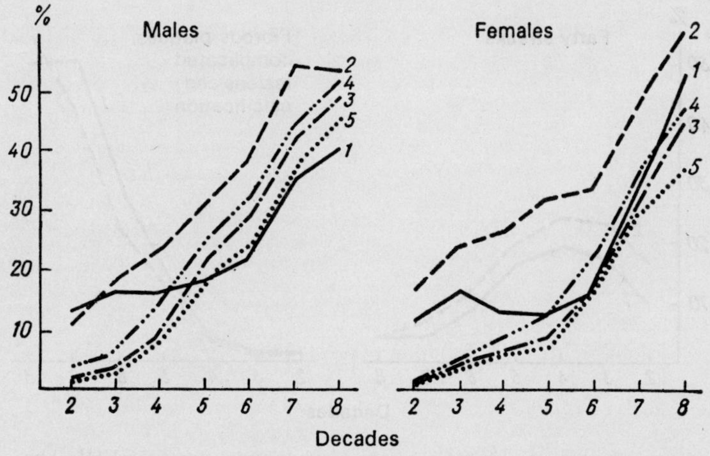

Figure 2. Total area of atherosclerotic changes in vessels of EHI. The ordinate shows the total area of arteriosclerotic changes expressed as percentage of intimal surface of vessels. Curve *1*, thoracic aorta; *2*, abdominal aorta; *3*, right coronary artery; *4*, LAD coronary artery; *5*, left circumflex coronary artery.

Variations in the types of atherosclerotic changes have also been observed. The area occupied by fatty streaks in both parts of the aorta of males and females increases with age up to the fourth decade of life. At that time it reaches a maximum in the abdominal aorta, occupying 20–25% of the intimal surface. Then the area of lipidosis gradually decreases, and in the eighth decade of life it involves 3–4% of the intimal surface. In the abdominal aorta the area occupied by fatty streaks in all age groups was considerably higher in females than in males. In coronary arteries the area occupied by fatty streaks was less than in the aorta, and occupied less than 4–5% of the intimal surface in all the age groups. Mean values of the areas with lipidosis were higher in females than in males, although the differences were not always significant (Figs. 3 and 4).

In the aorta and coronary arteries, there are considerable differences in the dynamics of lipidosis: in the aorta the area with fatty streaks increases up to the fourth decade of life and then gradually decreases; in the coronary arteries the area of lipidosis is more or less constant, i.e., no change is observed throughout the subject's life (Fig. 5).

In all vessels, fibrous plaques appear in the second decade of life. With age, the area affected with these lesions gradually increases, and in the eighth decade they occupy 40–45% of the intimal surface of the aorta and 35–40% of the intimal surface of the coronary arteries (Table 5; Fig. 5). It should be noted that the area with fibrous plaques increases considerably in the first few decades of life. Later the rate of growth of fibrous plaques gradually

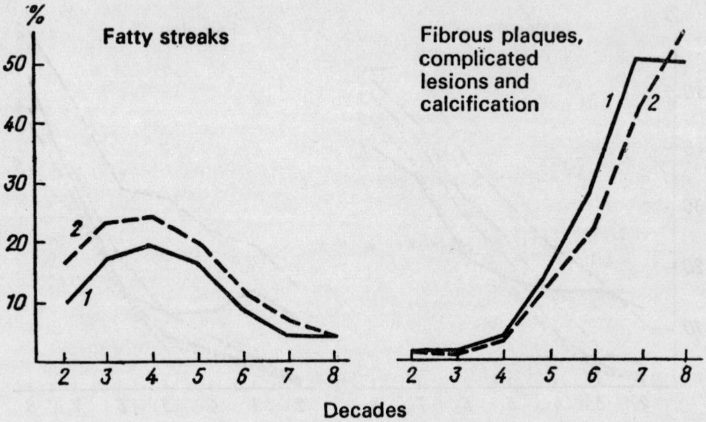

Figure 3. Atherosclerotic changes in abdominal aorta of EHI. The ordinate shows the changed area as a percentage of intimal surface of vessel. Curve *1*, males; *2*, females.

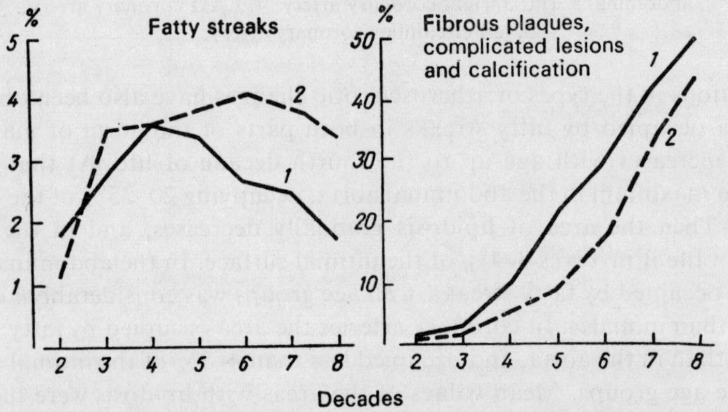

Figure 4. Atherosclerotic changes in the LAD coronary artery of EHI. The ordinate shows the changed area as a percentage of intimal surface of the vessel. Curve *1*, males; *2*, females.

decreases. Compared with previous decades, the area of fibrous plaques increases 3 to 4 times in the fourth and fifth decades of life, 1.5 to 2 times in the sixth and seventh decades and only 1.2 to 1.3 times in the eighth decade.

Fibrous plaques in both parts of aorta occupied a somewhat larger area in males up to the eighth decade but appeared in females only in the eighth decade. In coronary arteries the extent of fibrous plaques in males was always greater than in females, and the differences usually were statistically significant (see Table 5).

Complicated lesions (plaques with hemorrhages, erosions, thrombosis)

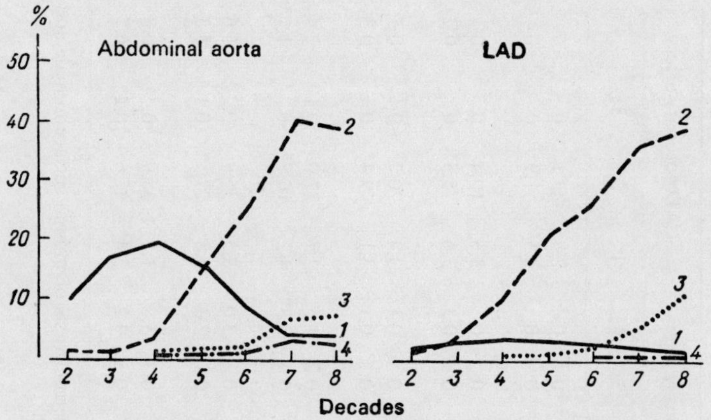

Figure 5. Characteristics of development of various types of atherosclerotic changes in the abdominal aorta of male EHIs. Ordinate shows the changed area as a percentage of intimal surface of the vessel. Curve *1*, fatty streaks; *2*, fibrous plaques; *3*, calcification; *4*, complicated lesions.

appear in males and females in the fourth decade of life. They are noticed more frequently in the abdominal aorta, where the area with these lesions is maximal in the eighth decade of life (on an average about 3% of the area of a vessel). In coronary arteries the lesion area similarly increases with age, but even in older age groups it averages not more than 0.5% of the area of a vessel. Complicated lesions were more widely distributed in all the vessels of males than of females; in the aorta these differences were often statistically significant (Table 5).

Calcification was noticed from the fourth decade of life in the vessels studied. The area occupied by calcified plaques steadily increases with age and by the eighth decade reaches 2–3% in the thoracic aorta, 7–9% in the abdominal aorta, and about 11% in the LAD coronary artery in males and 7% in females.

The area with calcification in both parts of the aorta was somewhat greater in males up to 70 years and in females aged more than 70; in the coronary arteries of all age groups the area with calcification was greater in males. It was noticed that the differences between males and females were very rarely statistically significant (Table 5).

An analysis of the different types of atherosclerotic changes demonstrates that in subjects up to 40 years of age the total area of atherosclerotic changes was mainly because of lipidosis, which considerably exceeded the area with fibrous plaques. In older age groups the share of fibrous plaques of the total area becomes still greater; from the sixth decade of life it becomes predominant. The variations in the rate of development of lipidosis and fibrous plaques in the aorta and coronary arteries deserve attention.

Table 5. Average Area of Atherosclerotic Changes in the Aorta and Coronary Arteries

Age in years	Sex	Thoracic aorta				Abdominal aorta				Right coronary artery				LAD coronary artery			
		1†	2	3	4	1	2	3	4	1	2	3	4	1	2	3	4
20–29	Male	15.6	0.4	0	0	17.1	0.8	0	0	2.1	1.5	0	0	2.8	3.1	0	0
	Female	16.5	0.4	0	0	23.2*	0.9	0	0	3.2	1.0	0	0	3.5	1.9*	0	0
30–39	Male	14.8	1.3	0	0	19.5	3.6	0.1	0.1	4.5	4.5	0	0	3.6	10.4	0	0.1
	Female	12.3*	1.2	0	0	24.1*	2.9	0.1	0.1	2.8*	2.9*	0	0.3	3.6	5.5*	0	0.2
40–49	Male	12.0	5.2	0.3	0.1	16.4	14.0	0.2	0.4	4.4	16.4	0	0.1	3.4	20.7	0	0.5
	Female	8.0*	4.0	0	0	19.9*	11.9	0.1	0.3	3.4	5.8*	0	0.1	3.1	9.4*	0	0.3
50–59	Male	7.2	14.4	0.3	0.2	9.0	25.8	1.4	1.5	4.5	22.7	0.2	1.5	2.7	27.0	0.1	2.4
	Female	6.3	10.6*	0.1	0.1	11.9*	20.8*	0.4*	1.1	5.0	11.4*	0.4	0.3*	4.2	16.7*	0	1.1*
60–69	Male	4.7	28.4	1.0	1.1	4.0	40.7	3.3	6.2	3.7	34.1	0.3	3.0	2.5	35.9	0.2	5.6
	Female	5.5	26.5	0.5	1.1	6.7*	36.5	1.3*	3.9*	5.4*	25.0*	0.1	2.3	3.8	27.5*	0.1	5.3
70–79	Male	3.0	33.6	2.0	2.0	4.0	39.7	2.9	7.2	1.8	41.2	0.3	5.8	1.7	38.9	0.5	10.8
	Female	4.3*	42.1*	1.2	3.0	4.3	45.1	1.9	8.7	4.5*	36.7	0.3	3.2	3.4*	37.6	0.2*	6.7

* Statistically significant differences ($p \leqslant 0.05$) between the indices showing the percentage of atherosclerosis of intimal surface in male and female EHI.

† Stage 1, lipid streaks; 2, fibrous plaques; 3, complicated lesions; 4, calcification.

Lipidosis occupies a greater area in the aorta of young persons, but with age there is a very rapid decrease in its area; in the coronary arteries the average area of lipidosis is very extensive and changes insignificantly with age. In spite of this the rates of development of fibrous plaques both in the aorta and in coronary arteries were more or less the same. The rates of development of fibrous plaques in the abdominal aorta are similar to the rates of development in the LAD coronary artery and development in the thoracic aorta is similar to the rate in the remaining coronary arteries. While lipidosis in the aorta and coronary arteries is usually more marked in females than in males, the development of fibrous plaques in males takes place at a more rapid rate, particularly in the coronary arteries. From these data it may be gathered that there is no direct relationship between the degree of lipidosis and the rate and degree of development of fibrous plaques. Our data confirm the opinion of several authors (Anichkov, 1947; Davydovskii, 1967) that fatty streaks may disappear to a considerable extent and not undergo sclerotic changes. Since fatty streaks, even when they occupy a considerable part of the intima of a vessel, do not determine the severity of atherosclerosis, the characterization of atherosclerosis should be based on both the total area of atherosclerotic changes and on the total area with fibrous plaques, complicated lesions, and calcification (the changes defined as raised lesions by the working group of WHO pathologists).

Our data showing the dynamics of lipidosis in the aorta (a decrease in the area of lipidosis with age) coincide with the data of Holman *et al.* (1958), Strong and McGill (1969), Alekseev (1968), and others. However, a study of aortas not stained with Sudan (Avtandilov, 1970) showed different results—a continuous rise in the area of lipidosis with age. These variations are probably due to the imperfect methods of examination Avtandilov used, since an evaluation of lipidosis in unstained specimens lacks accuracy. Moreover, it is not unlikely that the concept of lipidosis as understood by Avtandilov was somewhat different from that of the study group of WHO pathologists. The WHO study group defined lipidosis as the accumulation of lipids only in an unchanged intima; during macroscopic examination of vessels it is not possible to determine the thickness of the intima by palpation.

Study of the rates of development of atherosclerotic changes showed considerable non-uniformity in the advancement of atherosclerosis with age. This was noticed both during study of the total area of atherosclerotic changes and in different types of lesions. The rates of development of raised lesions with age hold special interest because it is mainly these lesions that determine the severity of atherosclerosis. According to our data, in both parts of the aorta of males and females a maximal rise in the area with raised lesions was noticed in the fifth decade of life; the increase in the lesion area compared with the previous decade of life was more than threefold. In the subsequent decades the rate of growth decreased, and in the eighth decade of life the area showing the changes increased only by 1.2 to 1.3 times. Such rates of increase in the total area with fibrous plaques, complicated lesions, and calcification were noted in the coronary arteries of males. In females the growth rate was more or less equal in the fifth, sixth, and seventh decades, but in all the vessels it was minimal in the eighth decade of life. Several other workers also noticed a non-uniform progression of atherosclerosis with age. According to the findings of White *et al.* (1950) the rates of development of coronary atherosclerosis were greatest in males between 30 and 49 years. In his study Avtandilov (1965, 1970) noted that the increase in the area with atherosclerotic lesions in the aorta and coronary arteries was in geometric progression with each succeeding decade of life (in the aorta, 2 times; in the right coronary artery, 1.8 times; in the left coronary artery, 1.6 times). These discrepancies in the evaluation of the rates of progression of the atherosclerotic process reflect the methodical characteristics of the work of Avtandilov, who analyzed the materials without dividing according to sex and examined unstained vessels.

It is necessary to emphasize that the data as we present them, like the observations of other investigators, show that the progression of atherosclerosis in various vessels and in subjects of different sex has its individual characteristics. One should pay attention to the fact that atherosclerotic changes take place unevenly throughout life, and after 70 years of age the development of atherosclerosis is sharply retarded.

CHARACTERISTICS OF THE DEVELOPMENT OF ATHEROSCLEROSIS IN EHI AND OBESITY

The interrelationship between the degree of obesity and the development of atherosclerosis in man has long attracted the attention of scientists and has been discussed very thoroughly in the literature. As the degree of obesity in man to a certain extent is determined by the type of nutrition, a study of the present problem in relation to the role of alimentary factors in the pathogenesis of atherosclerosis is of interest. Also it is well known that an increase in weight, particularly a rapid increase in body weight after 25 years, is considered to be one of the risk factors for coronary heart disease and especially for myocardial infarction (Ashley and Kannel, 1974).

However, in the literature the available data showing the characteristic of atherosclerosis in people with various types of nutrition are contradictory (Volkova, 1946; Pronin, 1961; Myasnikov, 1965; Giertsen, 1966; Montenegro and Solberg, 1968; Sternby, 1968). The discrepancy in the pathological data partly reflects the considerable change in the type of nutrition of the patients because of the principal disease and because of the selection of cases in the terminal stage and the great diversity of the groups being compared.

Different indices are used to characterize the type of nutrition: body weight, the relation between height and body weight, the thickness of subcutaneous fatty tissue. Sternby (1968) conducted a comparative study to correlate these indices with the degree of atherosclerosis in various vessels and concluded that any of these indices may be used for the same purpose as long as they give similar results.

A group of EHIs is most suitable for studying the present problem since they demonstrate some stability in the type of nutrition compared with people who died from various diseases, and since use of the group practically excludes the effect of various diseases on the manifestation of atherosclerosis.

To judge the status of nutrition we considered the thickness of the subcutaneous fatty tissue in a standard place—a point midway between the umbilicus and the xiphoid process; this criterion has been utilized by other authors (Bjurulf, 1964; Montenegro and Solberg, 1968; Sternby, 1968; Möttönen, 1969). On the basis of the thickness of the subcutaneous fatty tissue in this location subjects were divided into two classes: (1) those with tissue thickness less than or equal to 20 mm in males and 25 mm in females were included in subgroup I; (2) those with tissue thickness greater than 20 mm in males and 25 mm in females were included in subgroup II. Data showing the mean thickness of the tissue in comparable subgroups is presented in Table 6. As can be seen from Table 6, the thickness of the tissue in subgroup II was more than double than that in I ($p \leqslant 0.001$).

Table 6. Mean Thickness of Subcutaneous Fatty Tissue in Healthy Lean (1) and Obese (2) EHI

Age in years	Subgroups	Males	Females
40–49	1	13.1 ± 0.2 (290)*	15.5 ± 0.7 (66)
	2	30.5 ± 1.3 (32)	41.9 ± 1.5 (43)
50–59	1	12.0 ± 0.3 (236)	17.1 ± 0.6 (78)
	2	27.5 ± 1.5 (27)	47.7 ± 1.2 (34)
60–69	1	12.9 ± 0.3 (138)	15.0 ± 0.8 (60)
	2	31.3 ± 1.7 (29)	35.6 ± 1.1 (33)

* Number of cases.

The distribution of males and females in the subgroups was not uniform: the number of males was considerably higher in subgroup I (664) than in II (88); in females distribution was more uniform between subgroup I (204) and subgroup II (110), i.e., among females obese individuals are more numerous. No significant variation in the prevalence of different types of atherosclerotic changes in the vessels studied was noted among the subgroups.

While analyzing the manifestation of atherosclerosis in EHI, depending on the degree of their obesity, clear sex-dependent differences were noted. In males the total area of atherosclerotic changes and the total area with raised lesions in the aorta were the same in the two comparable subgroups. However, in the coronary arteries the degree of atherosclerosis was considerably greater in obese subjects. In obese females the total area of atherosclerosis and the total area with raised lesions in all the vessels studied were usually less than in males (1). The difference is statistically significant (Table 7).

Table 7. Age-standardized (40–69 years) Indices of Diseased Areas in the Aorta and Coronary Arteries

Type of changes	Subgroups	ThA	AA	RCA	LADCA	LCCA
Males						
Lipidosis	1	8.1	9.5	4.3	2.9	3.5
	2	8.2	9.0	4.4	3.3	3.6
Raised lesions	1	16.5	29.4	25.5	29.0	21.9
	2	16.5	28.6	30.3*	33.5*	27.2*
Females						
Lipidosis	1	6.9	12.4	5.4	3.8	4.9
	2	7.0	15.9*	4.2	3.7	4.4
Raised lesions	1	16.8	29.4	16.6	23.4	16.3
	2	12.2*	23.5*	13.4	18.5*	10.0*

Vessels: ThA, thoracic aorta; AA, abdominal aorta; RCA, right coronary artery; LADCA, LAD coronary artery; LCCA, left circumflex coronary artery. Damage is a percentage of vessel intimal surface in lean (1) and obese (2) EHI.

* Differences were statistically significant ($p \leqslant 0.05$).

The extent of atherosclerotic changes in the vessels of people differed with the degree of obesity. Our attention is drawn to the fact that the area with lipidosis both in obese and in lean subjects was more or less the same. Only in certain decades of life do fatty streaks occupy a substantially greater area in the abdominal aorta of obese subjects; in females substantial differences in fatty streaks were observed in the abdominal aorta in age-standardized indices (Table 7).

The subgroup differences in the extent of fibrous plaques in vessels are similar to the subgroup differences in raised lesion areas. In both parts of the aorta in males the extent of fibrous plaques was the same, but in coronary arteries it was considerably greater in obese subjects, particularly in the age group between 40 and 49 years. In lean females the extent of fibrous plaques in all the vessels was greater, as compared to obese subjects. The extent of complicated lesions in the aorta and coronary arteries in the comparable subgroups was uniform.

The presence of severe calcification both in the aorta and in the coronary arteries of lean males and females was an unexpected finding. Here the differences were always unidirectional in nature and some of the comparisons were statistically significant. Earlier we observed (Vikhert *et al.*, 1967; Zhdanov, 1973) that in diseases associated with emaciation (cirrhosis of the liver, chronic pneumonia, chronic pulmonary tuberculosis) there is a tendency to intensified calcification in the aorta and coronary arteries, although the manifestation of other types of atherosclerotic changes is less compared with a control group. These data show that there is some peculiarity in the development of calcification in the vessels and that it is not directly dependent on the development of lipidosis and fibrous plaques. The biochemical findings of Eilerson and Faber (1960) also support this hypothesis. The authors emphasized that in pulmonary tuberculosis the deposition of calcium continues, although they observed a decrease in the accumulation of cholesterol in aorta.

The total area with raised lesions and fibrous plaques was compared in subjects in the obese subgroup and in those in the lean subgroup with fatty tissue not more than 10 mm thick (males with fatty tissue 11–20 mm thick and females with a tissue thickness of 11–25 mm were excluded from this comparison). Comparison of the subgroups supported our main findings. The differences between the subgroups, as was expected, remained practically the same.

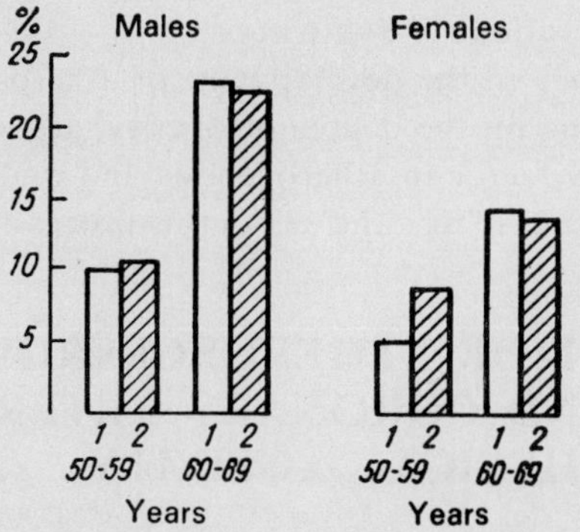

Figure 6. Prevalence of stenosis of coronary arteries (50% or more of lumen) in EHI with varying thickness of subcutaneous fatty tissue: White columns, subcutaneous fatty tissue less than 20 mm in males and 25 mm in females; shaded columns, subcutaneous fatty tissue more than 20 mm in males and 25 mm in females.

Stenosis of coronary arteries (more than 50% of their lumen) in males and females in comparable subgroups was noted only in the age groups between 50 and 59 and between 60 and 69 years. Here no significant differences were observed between the subgroups (Fig. 6). After analyzing 3174 autopsies

Sternby *et al.* (1965) were also unable to find any dependence between the thickness of the subcutaneous fatty tissue in an abdominal wall and stenosis of coronary arteries.

The data presented demonstrate that in the coronary arteries of obese males there is a more rapid development of atherosclerosis, as compared to lean males. This is evident from the materials showing the total area with atherosclerosis, the total area with raised lesions, and the area with fibrous plaques. The differences in the manifestation of atherosclerosis in the aorta of males were in fact absent in comparable subgroups. In obese females the manifestation of atherosclerosis was less in the aorta and in the coronary arteries.

Other workers have also shown diverse tendencies in the development of atherosclerosis in obese males and females. Henschen (1961) and Moses (1963) noted a relationship between the development of atherosclerosis and the degree of nutrition only in males. According to them, the degree of nutrition did not influence the degree of atherosclerosis in females.

In this connection it must be noted that obesity in males is often also associated with an increased muscle mass as compared to that of females. According to Spain *et al.* (1963) an increased muscle mass in association with obesity predisposes the individual to the development of coronary heart disease to a greater extent than obesity alone. Bjurulf (1964) to some extent supported these observations of Spain *et al.*

The varying tendency in the development of atherosclerosis in EH males and females, depending on the degree of obesity, argues against the leading role of the alimentary factor in atherogenesis and underlines the important role of the characteristics of age and sex in this process.

DEVELOPMENT OF ATHEROSCLEROSIS IN THE AORTA AND CORONARY ARTERIES IN EHI AND PHYSICAL ACTIVITY

Clinical and epidemiological studies demonstrate that coronary heart disease and essential hypertension are observed more in subjects engaged in "mental" work than in subjects engaged in physical work (Glazunov, 1961; Myasnikov, 1965; Ryvkin, 1965; Sedov, 1966; Novikov *et al.*, 1967; Frank, 1968; Fox and Paul, 1969; Simborg, 1970; Chazov *et al.*, 1972; Stamler *et al.*, 1972). In all probability this is because of inadequate physical activity and the psycho-emotional strain of these subjects (Shkhvatsabaya, 1964). The importance of the professional factor in the development of atherosclerosis is not clear.

The pathological data showing the nature and the rates of development of atherosclerosis in people performing various types of work are not very extensive. As a rule they are based on the study of groups of people dead from various diseases (Rapoport, 1935; Sedov, 1965) that in their own way influence the development of atherosclerosis (Vikhert *et al.*, 1967; Zhdanov, 1969). In this connection the study of atherosclerosis in EHI and its relation to the nature of their work would be of interest.

For this purpose we studied the coronary arteries and aortas of 430 EH males who had died between the ages of 40 and 60. An analysis of the corresponding groups of females was not undertaken because of the inadequate number of subjects engaged in "mental" work.

The cases were divided into two groups depending on the nature of their work. The first group consisted of 341 males engaged in physical work (industrial and construction workers, loaders, carpenters, smiths, and other types of workers); the second group consisted of 89 males engaged in mental work (accountants, administrative and scientific workers, doctors, engineers, and teachers). Drivers, who are engaged in a type of work having special characteristics, were not included in the groups studied. The difference between the groups was considered statistically significant when $p \leqslant 0.05$.

Significant differences were noted in the vessels studied according to the stage of atherosclerosis. In subjects engaged in physical work the vessels were often normal or showed only fatty streaks; in subjects engaged in mental work the vessels showed more severe stages of atherosclerosis, especially raised lesions (fibrous plaques, complicated lesions, and calcification).

The differences between the groups were statistically significant in the abdominal aorta, right coronary artery, and LAD coronary artery (Table 8).

Table 8. Age-standardized (40–69 years) Indices Showing Prevalence of Diseased Vessels in Subjects Performing Physical (1) and Mental (2) Work

Nature of changes	Subgroups	ThA	AA	RCA	LADCA	LCCA
Lipidosis	1	18.2	8.4	24.6	8.2	22.1
	2	17.6	1.3*	15.8*	3.4*	21.5
Raised lesions	1	81.8	91.6	75.4	91.8	77.9
	2	82.4	98.7*	84.2*	96.6*	78.5

ThA, thoracic aorta; AA, abdominal aorta; RCA, right coronary artery; LADCA, LAD coronary artery; LCCA, left circumflex coronary artery. Disease expressed as a percentage of vessel intimal surface.

* Statistically significant differences between groups ($p \leqslant 0.05$).

The most severe stages of atherosclerosis, i.e., vessels with complicated lesions and calcification, were also often noted in subjects doing mental work (in 11 out of the 15 compared), but these differences were not statistically significant.

A comparison of the groups studied in respect to the area or the extent of atherosclerotic changes in the aorta and coronary arteries demonstrated certain differences between them. In all the vessels the total area with atherosclerotic changes, the area with raised lesions (fibrous plaques, complicated lesions, and calcification), and the area with fibrous plaques (in the fourth, fifth, and sixth decades of life) were greater in subjects engaged in mental work (Fig. 7 and Table 9). The differences between the groups in the extent of these changes in both parts of the aorta were somewhat less than the extent of these lesions in the coronary arteries. In the age-standardized (40–69 years) indices of the area with fibrous plaques, the total area with raised lesions for all the vessels (except the abdominal aorta) was considerably greater in subjects performing mental work.

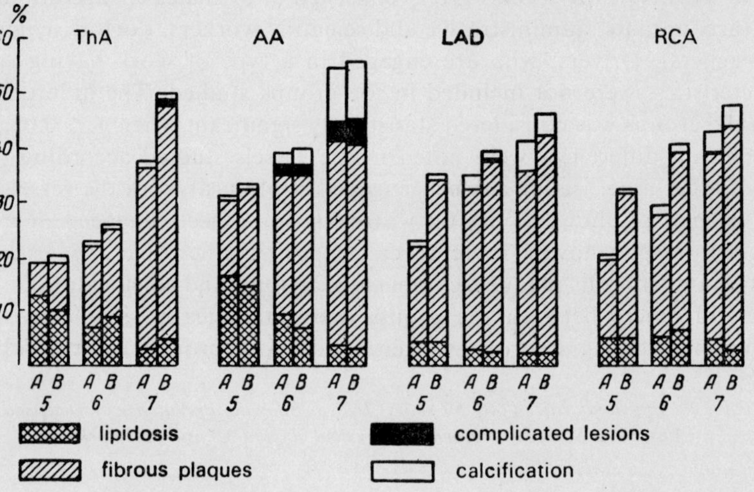

Figure 7. The nature of atherosclerosis in vessels of EH males engaged in physical (*A*) and mental (*B*) work. Ordinate, percentage of changed area in relation to intimal surface of vessels; abscissa, decades of life.

For other types of atherosclerotic changes, particularly fatty streaks, complicated lesions, and calcification, statistically significant differences were not noted between the groups.

Stenosis of coronary arteries in those between 40 and 49 years and between 60 and 69 years in the two comparable groups were often practically the same (in the 40 to 49 age group, stenosis was seen in 2.4–2.8% of cases and in the 60 to 69 age group, in 24.2% of cases). In the 50 to 59 age group stenosis was noted more in subjects performing mental work (20%) than in subjects doing physical work (12.9%).

Thus the data indicate that atherosclerosis in the aorta and coronary arteries of EHI depends on the nature of the work and that clear-cut differences exist between manual and mental workers. The data show that in subjects performing mental work atherosclerosis is more marked, which indicates that in this group the rate of development is much more rapid. Marked atherosclerosis of the coronary arteries in intellectuals is probably one of the important causes of their greater rate of heart attacks.

Table 9. Age-standardized (40–69 years) Indices of Diseased Areas in the Aorta and Coronary Arteries in Subjects Performing Physical (1) and Mental (2) Work

Nature of changes	Subgroups	ThA	AA	RCA	LADCA	LCCA
Lipidosis	1	7.5	9.5	4.4	2.7	3.7
	2	7.8	7.9	4.4	2.8	3.4
Raised lesions	1	18.5	31.9	26.2	30.1	22.4
	2	23.8*	34.8	35.7*	40.5*	30.3*

ThA, thoracic aorta; AA, abdominal aorta; RCA, right coronary artery; LADCA, LAD coronary artery; LCCA, left circumflex coronary artery. Areas expressed as percentage of intimal surface.

* Differences between groups are statistically significant ($p \leqslant 0.05$).

The data in the present work showing the more rapid development of atherosclerosis in subjects performing mental work are in agreement with the results of biochemical tests of lipid metabolism on EHI according to profession. The blood cholesterol level was higher in subjects performing mental work (Myasnikov, 1965; Sedov, 1966), and among professional workers the cholesterol level was highest in those whose work was connected with considerable nervous strain.

Though there were differences in the blood cholesterol level in subjects performing physical or mental work, the area with lipidosis in the aorta and coronary arteries, according to our findings, was practically the same in the comparable groups. This probably results from the more rapid development of fibrous plaques in the vessels of subjects performing mental work in the presence of a high blood cholesterol level.

CONCLUSIONS

In the second decade of life, in nearly 99–100% of cases in both parts of the aorta of EHI, there are fatty streaks and fibrous plaques. Complicated lesions and calcification appear in the subsequent decades of life. Beginning with the fifth decade in the thoracic aorta and with the fourth in the abdominal aorta, complicated lesions are noted in most cases.

In contrast to the aorta, the coronary arteries, in the second to fourth decades of life in the majority of EHI (especially in females), show no macroscopic signs of atherosclerosis. Along with this, it must be noted that the tendency for the development of fibrous changes in the coronary arteries is greater than in the aorta. The significant differences in the prevalence of fibrous plaques (atherosclerosis stage II) in the aorta and coronary arteries testify to this. Males in the second decade of life had fibrous plaques in the abdominal aorta in 7.3% of cases, 20% in the third decade, and 53.6% in the fourth. In the LAD coronary artery, however, they were noted more frequently in 18.1%, 48.1%, and 68.5% of the cases, respectively.

In the aorta and coronary arteries the area with atherosclerotic changes, other than fatty streaks, increases with age. The area with lipidosis in the aorta increases with age only up to the third or fourth decade of life (occupying up to 25% of the intimal surface in the abdominal aorta); then the area with fatty streaks gradually decreases, and by the eighth or ninth decade usually occupies not more than 4–5% of the intimal surface of the aorta. In the coronary arteries the main area with lipidosis changes little with age. In people of various age groups lipidosis occupies approximately 3–5% of the area of the intimal surface. In females the extent of fatty streaks was greater than in males.

The total area with raised lesions (fibrous plaques, complicated lesions, and calcification) in the aorta occupied a somewhat greater area in males up to the eighth decade of life; however, the changes were more prevalent in females more than 70 years of age. In the coronary arteries raised lesions occupied a significantly greater area in males than in females; the differences between the sexes were due to the variation in the extent of fibrous plaques and, to a smaller degree, to differences in complicated lesions and calcification in coronary arteries of males and females. Atherosclerotic changes do not develop uniformly throughout life. A maximum growth of raised lesions, mostly of fibrous plaques, is often observed in the fifth decade of life; after 70 years of age there is a sharp retardation in the development of atherosclerosis in the vessels studied.

In essentially healthy obese males more signs indicating a high degree of atherosclerosis are often observed in the coronary arteries (complicated lesions, the total area with raised lesions, the area with fibrous plaques) than in lean subjects. The degree of nutrition does not influence the development of atherosclerosis in the aorta of males. In practically healthy obese females a reverse tendency was noticed: the development of atherosclerosis was considerably less in the abdominal aorta and coronary arteries than in lean females.

There were considerable variations in the manifestation of atherosclerosis, especially in the coronary arteries of EHI, depending on the nature of their work. The degree of atherosclerosis in the vessels studied was more severe in subjects performing mental work, and in these vessels the extent of raised lesions was greater; there were no differences between the groups in the area of the vessels with lipidosis.

The data in the present work and from other studies show considerable individual variations in the degree of atherosclerosis even when the group is homogeneous with regard to sex, age, and causes of death.

These variations undoubtedly indicate that the development of atherosclerosis in man is determined not by one but by several factors. Moreover, when studying the effect of various known risk factors on the course of atherosclerosis in man, it was apparent that there are probably many unknown factors. The groups of EHI and especially the subgroups (divisions were made considering the risk factors for ischemic heart disease and atherosclerosis) are without any doubt quite adequate for studying the factors favoring or retarding the development of atherosclerosis.

2

Atherosclerosis as a Primary Disease

The study of the age-related dynamics, the rate of development and the qualitative characteristics of the atherosclerotic process in those for whom the cause of death is directly related to atherosclerosis or, more precisely, to its complications, is particularly interesting. This group characterizes the progressive development of atherosclerotic changes that are responsible for the development of myocardial infarction, cardiosclerosis (ischemic cardiomyopathy), cerebrovascular strokes, and others. In recent years there has been a tendency to consider the main complications of atherosclerosis as independent nosological entities. Ischemic heart disease was an independent nosological entity in the international statistical classification of diseases, traumas, and the causes of death. This classification was introduced in the USSR on January 1, 1970. But we will use the term "coronary disease," because it reflects the disease more completely; atherosclerotic lesions of the coronary arteries are the basis for the development and subsequent progression of the disease. It should be noted that different changes in organs like the heart, brain, and lower extremities are usually observed in severe stages of atherosclerosis. Diagnosis of coronary heart disease in most cases is synonymous with the diagnosis of atherosclerosis of the coronary arteries, leading to stenosis, with or without thrombosis, accompanied by myocardial infarction and often followed by cardiosclerosis.

Many investigators have studied the vascular changes in persons dying from the complications of atherosclerosis. However, most studies have been based exclusively on the analysis of autopsy records. Only in the last 10 years have morphological studies of the atherosclerotic process been reported for this group of people. As expected, the studies showed that in patients dying from the complications of atherosclerosis the development of atherosclerotic changes takes place at a more rapid rate than in other individuals.

Avtandilov (1965, 1970) subdivides his own cases into three main groups: healthy, patients with atherosclerosis, and patients with other diseases. In those dying from atherosclerosis the development of atherosclerotic changes is characterized as "accelerated," in the healthy as "retarded," in others as "intermediate." On the basis of biochemical tests of the vessels Giertsen (1966) came to the conclusion that subjects with atherosclerotic heart disease have more severe atherosclerosis than other patients, except patients belonging to a very old age group. This was also noted by Vanecek *et al.* (1967), who found considerably more extensive changes in the abdominal aorta and coronary arteries of patients dying from atherosclerosis than of subjects belonging to other groups.

A large number of investigators have presented data showing the nature of atherosclerotic changes in the coronary arteries in patients with ischemic heart disease (primarily patients with myocardial infarction) (Sedov, 1965; Giertsen, 1966; Vikhert and Matova, 1967; Sternby, 1968).

In our studies those dead from complications of atherosclerosis, as well as the group of EHI, constituted the two main control groups for characterizing atherosclerosis in persons dying from various diseases. The group comprising persons dying from complications of atherosclerosis included subjects dying from myocardial infarction, acute and chronic coronary insufficiency, cerebrovascular accidents, gangrene of the lower extremities, and gangrene of the intestines due to atherosclerotic lesions of the mesenteric arteries. Based on the materials available from the case histories and the autopsy results, the development of complications noted above was attributed to atherosclerosis by a pathologist or by a specialist in forensic medicine. Those suffering from hypertension, diabetes mellitus, and other chronic diseases that could affect the development of atherosclerosis were not included in this group. To characterize the atherosclerotic process in this group, a morphological study of atherosclerosis was conducted with the aortas and coronary arteries of 837 persons dying from atherosclerosis (522 males and 315 females 40 to 79 years of age).

In both males and females dying from complications of atherosclerosis the different types of atherosclerotic changes were present in the aorta in 100% of cases; however, such changes were noted in EHI also. The differences between these groups existed: in the aorta of EHI fatty streaks and/or fibrous plaques were more often noted, but in those dying from atherosclerosis complicated lesions, calcification, or both were generally present. In particular major differences were noted in a group of EH males in the fifth and sixth decades and in females in the sixth and seventh decades of life; in the subsequent years (the seventh and eighth in males and the eighth decade of life in females) the differences between the above groups diminished (Table 10). Among males calcification was seen more frequently in those dying from atherosclerosis only in the fifth and sixth decades of life, but in females the difference was present in these decades and in the seventh decade; in the subsequent decades of life the differences between the groups were insignificant. In subjects dying from atherosclerosis in the fifth decade of life calcification

*Table 10. Prevalence of Atherosclerotic Stages in EHI (1) and in Subjects Dying from Atherosclerosis (2)**

Age in years	Subgroups	Abdominal aorta			Right coronary artery			LAD coronary artery		
		0–I	II	III–IV	0–I	II	III–IV	0–I	II	III–IV
Males										
40–49	1	15.4	65.0	19.6	32.5	61.2	7.3	13.3	75.8	10.9
	2	9.1	38.9	52.0	13.9	52.8	33.3	4.2	43.0	52.8
50–59	1	7.3	46.4	46.3	17.8	61.9	20.3	7.3	65.5	27.2
	2	0	26.7	73.3	8.2	52.5	39.3	3.3	36.7	60.0
60–69	1	2.0	21.5	76.5	7.7	54.5	37.8	2.8	52.5	44.7
	2	1.8	11.0	87.2	2.4	35.6	62.0	0.7	22.5	76.8
70–79	1	1.4	14.1	84.5	7.2	45.6	47.2	4.3	37.7	58.0
	2	0.7	8.2	91.1	3.5	35.2	61.3	1.4	25.4	73.2
Females										
50–59	1	9.4	56.2	35.4	39.7	46.2	16.1	19.8	59.3	20.9
	2	2.3	29.5	68.2	22.2	55.5	22.3	21.4	38.5	46.1
60–69	1	0	41.5	58.5	15.8	63.5	20.7	9.9	54.3	35.8
	2	0.8	20.7	78.5	6.0	56.4	37.6	4.5	35.1	60.4
70–79	1	0	20.7	79.3	5.9	51.0	47.1	2.0	36.0	62.0
	2	0	9.3	90.7	3.7	42.6	54.7	0	32.0	68.0

* Stage 0–I, vessels without changes or with only lipidosis; Stage II, vessels with only lipidosis and fibrous plaques; Stage III–IV, vessels with complicated lesions and/or calcification. Prevalence is expressed as a percentage of total observations.

was noted in 33.8% in the abdominal aorta; in the sixth, in 58.3%; in the seventh, in 67.4%; and in the eighth, in 77.4%. In healthy people calcification was present in 14.6%, 37.6%, 63.8%, and 78.7% of cases, respectively.

Complicated lesions are the most characteristic changes in the aorta of those dying from atherosclerosis; they were seen in these subjects more frequently than in healthy people. In the fifth decade of life, complicated lesions were noted in 41.6% of males dying from atherosclerosis and in only 11% of healthy individuals; in the eighth decade of life, the percentages were 82.9% and 61.4%, respectively.

Coronary arteries showed no changes, lipidosis only, or lipidosis and fibrous plaques more frequently in EHI; those dying from atherosclerosis showed complicated lesions and calcification more frequently (Table 10). Calcification of the coronary arteries was seen more frequently in those dying from atherosclerosis than in healthy individuals, but with an increase in age the differences between the groups declined somewhat. In males dying from atherosclerosis, calcification in the LAD coronary artery in the fifth decade of life was seen in 26.1%, in the sixth in 54%, in the seventh in 73.5%, and in the eighth in 71.1% cases; in healthy individuals calcification was present in 10.5%, 25.5%, 44%, and 53.7% of cases, respectively. In both groups calcification of the coronary arteries in the age groups up to 70 years was noted more in males than in females; in subjects above 70 years of age, differences between the sexes in the frequency of calcification in the groups were practically absent.

Complicated lesions were noted more rarely in coronary arteries than calcification, but the differences between the groups were always more significant for complicated lesions than for calcification; complicated lesions in subjects dying from atherosclerosis were often present threefold or more times than in healthy subjects.

In males dying from atherosclerosis complicated lesions in LAD coronary artery in the fifth decade of life were noted in 30.6%, in the sixth in 18.7%, in the seventh in 20.5%, and in the eighth in 14.8% of cases; in healthy subjects these were present in only 1.6%, 3.9%, 7.7%, and 5.8% of cases. The differences in the frequency of complicated lesions between these two groups were mainly due to thrombosis of the coronary arteries, found only in the group of patients dying from complications of atherosclerosis.

These data indicate that the typical atherosclerotic changes in the coronary arteries (and also in the aorta) of those who died from complications of atherosclerosis are calcification and complicated lesions.

Data showing the area and extent of atherosclerotic changes in subjects dying from complications of atherosclerosis are presented in Table 11 and in Figs. 8 and 9. The area showing these changes, except the area with lipidosis, in the vessels studied was greater in subjects dying from complications of atherosclerosis than in the healthy.

Table 11. Mean Area with Raised Lesions in Subjects Dying from Atherosclerosis

Age in years (number of cases)	Abdominal aorta			LAD coronary artery			Right coronary artery		
	FbPl*	Co	Ca	FbPl	Co	Ca	FbPl	Co	Ca
Males									
40–49 (77)	30.9	2.9	1.1	47.7	1.0	3.0	42.6	0.8	0.6
50–59 (173)	39.7	4.6	3.6	41.9	1.0	6.3	40.7	1.2	2.3
60–69 (189)	47.3	7.7	5.3	46.7	1.1	11.8	44.9	1.3	6.4
70–79 (78)	53.6	9.1	7.3	45.2	0.4	12.8	55.5	1.3	5.6
Females									
40–49 (19)	18.6	0.2	0.1	26.8	0	1.6	25.0	1.5	1.5
50–59 (47)	39.8	2.2	4.6	36.0	1.0	3.4	28.8	0.2	1.7
60–69 (150)	46.8	4.0	7.3	43.8	2.6	7.9	41.4	0.3	4.1
70–79 (105)	49.6	5.3	9.2	42.4	0.8	11.5	46.1	0.8	5.8

* FbPl, fibrous plaques; Co, complicated lesions; Ca, calcification. Disease expressed as a percentage of the intimal surface of the vessels.

The total area of atherosclerotic changes in all the vessels was always greater in subjects dying from complications of atherosclerosis than in EHI. Moreover, the differences between the groups were statistically significant in 38 out of the 40 comparisons made (five vessels, each compared in four age groups, separately for males and females).

The analysis revealed that only fatty streaks occupied a greater area in healthy people. Raised lesions (fibrous plaques, complicated lesions, and calcification) were always more frequent in subjects dying from the complications of atherosclerosis. The area with lipidosis was greater in EHI; in 21 out of 40 comparisons the difference in area with lipidosis was statistically significant. Substantial differences between the groups in the area with lipidosis are also apparent with an age-standardized index (40–79 years). In both parts of the aorta the area with lipidosis gradually decreases with age. The area with lipidosis was maximal in the abdominal aorta between 40 and 49 years in females dying from atherosclerosis. It was $18.7 \pm 2.3\%$ of the intimal surface (in males belonging to these ages, $11.0 \pm 1.3\%$); between 70 and 79 years the area occupied by lipidosis in both parts of the aorta in males and females was less than 4–5% of the intimal surface. In the coronary arteries the area with lipidosis in all the age groups was not high (3–5% of the intimal surface), and there was no marked variation with advancing age. The area with lipidosis in the LAD coronary artery was often somewhat less than in the right coronary artery and the left circumflex coronary artery.

The area with fibrous plaques increased with age in all the vessels both in

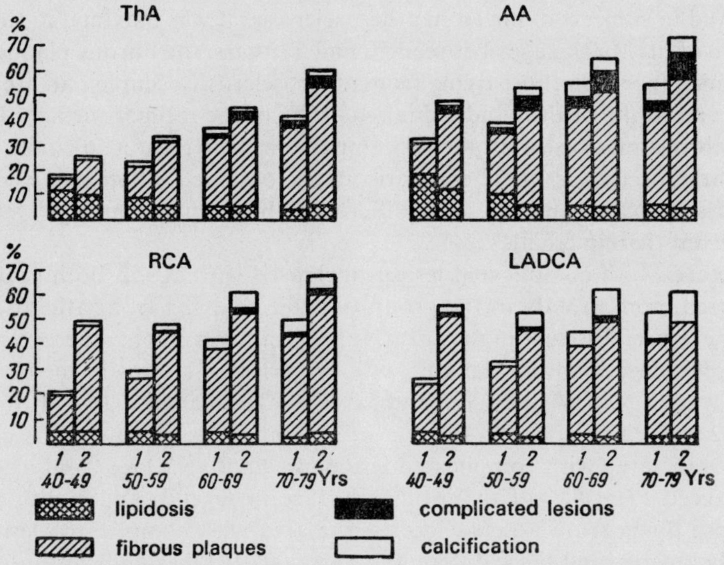

Figure 8. Dynamics of atherosclerotic changes of EHI (*1*) and of subjects dying from complications of atherosclerosis (*2*) in males. Percentage of changed area in respect to area of vessel is represented on the ordinate.

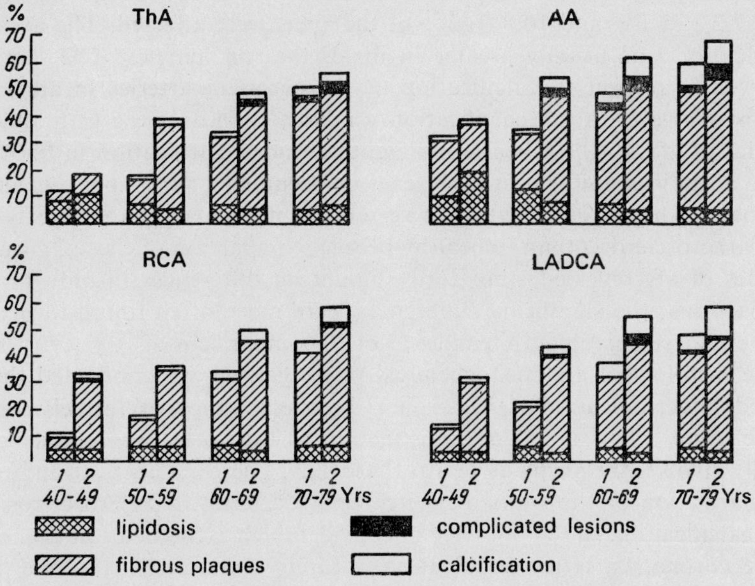

Figure 9. Dynamics of atherosclerotic changes of EHI (*1*) and of subjects dying from complications of atherosclerosis (*2*) in females.

EHI and in subjects dying from atherosclerosis; it was maximal in the eighth decade of life. In the ages between 70 and 79 years, the fibrous plaques in the abdominal aorta in those dying from atherosclerosis occupied an area of 50–53%, and in the healthy individual, 40–45% of the intimal surface. The area with fibrous plaques in all the 40 comparisons was greater in subjects dying from atherosclerosis; in 32 comparisons the observed differences were statistically significant. In males the differences between the groups were more significant than in females.

The area with complicated lesions increased with age in both groups, but increased more rapidly in the group of subjects dying from atherosclerosis; this was especially clear in the aorta. In subjects dying from atherosclerosis, in the eighth decade of life the area with complicated lesions in the abdominal aorta was $9.1 \pm 1.5\%$ in males and $5.3 \pm 1.2\%$ in females. In EHI the values were $2.9 \pm 0.5\%$ and $1.9 \pm 0.3\%$ of the intimal surface. In the coronary arteries the area with complicated lesions was not very great and usually did not exceed 1.0–1.5% of the intimal surface in seventh and eighth decades. In those dying from atherosclerosis, the area with complicated lesions was usually greater, and these differences were statistically significant in 24 out of 40 comparisons.

The area with calcification in all the vessels studied in both groups increased with age and was maximal in the eighth decade of life. In males dying from atherosclerosis, calcification was present in $7.3 \pm 1\%$ of the abdominal aorta and in $12.8 \pm 2.3\%$ of the intimal surface of the LAD coronary artery. In EHI, $7.2 \pm 1.1\%$ and $10.8 \pm 2\%$ of the areas were affected. The area with calcification was usually greater in males than in females. The same was observed in respect to calcification of the coronary arteries in all the age groups. However, aorta calcification was greater in only the fifth and sixth decades of life; in the seventh and eighth decades calcification in both parts of the aorta was uniform in both sexes or occupied a somewhat greater area in females. Though calcification of vessels was more marked in subjects dying from atherosclerosis than in healthy people, comparison of the subgroups by decades of life revealed statistically significant differences in only 11 of 40 comparisons; the significant differences were more often found in males (8 of 20 comparisons) than in females (3 of 20 comparisons).

The histological and histochemical investigations we conducted demonstrated that calcification of the coronary arteries is almost exclusively confined to the intima. This is in contradistinction to the aorta, where calcification usually involves the media as well as the intima. There is a correlation between vascularization of the walls of the coronary arteries in atherosclerosis and their calcification. In the presence of considerable vascularization of the walls of the coronary arteries calcification is rarely noted and, as a rule, is not marked. On the other hand, in the presence of extensive calcification of coronary arteries the vascularization of the walls was very slight (Fig. 10A, B).

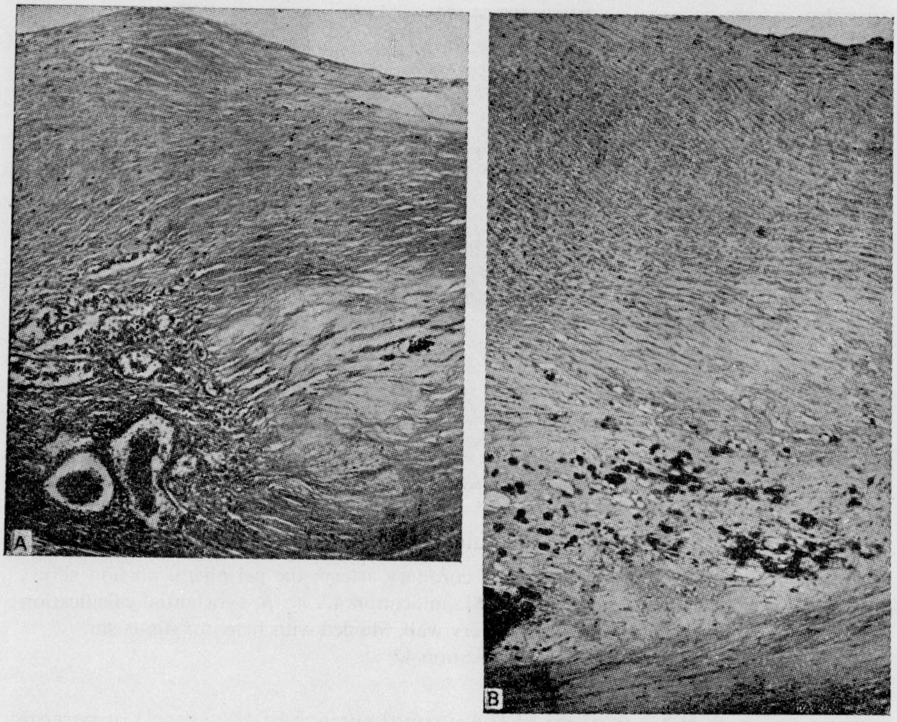

Figure 10. Characteristics of calcification of coronary arteries depending on the degree of vascularization of the abnormal vessel wall. *A*, marked vascularization of the sclerosed wall of a coronary artery with insignificant deposition of calcium salts (black granular masses on the right); *B*, considerable deposition of calcium salts in a poorly vascularized plaque. Stained with hematoxylin-eosin. Magnification 65 × 0.

Calcification of coronary arteries is more marked in formed plaques, i.e., in atherosclerotic plaques with well marked fibrous coverings and clear-cut boundaries between the atheromatous masses and neighboring vessel tissues. Deposition of calcium in coronary arteries in atherosclerosis is observed primarily along the periphery of an atheromatous lesion (mostly in the base). Fine granular deposits of calcium salts are most often noted in the media in the dystrophic area of the vessel wall. In addition, particularly in the presence of ischemic heart disease, a different type of calcification is often noted: extensive calcification of the necrotic parts of fibrous plaques may be present (Fig. 11). It is probable that the latter type of calcification rapidly produces extensive calcification of coronary arteries.

Subjects dying from various complications of atherosclerosis have greater areas with raised lesions than EHI when observations are compared by decades of life. This is supported by the data showing a greater frequency of severe degrees of atherosclerosis (cases in which the total area with raised

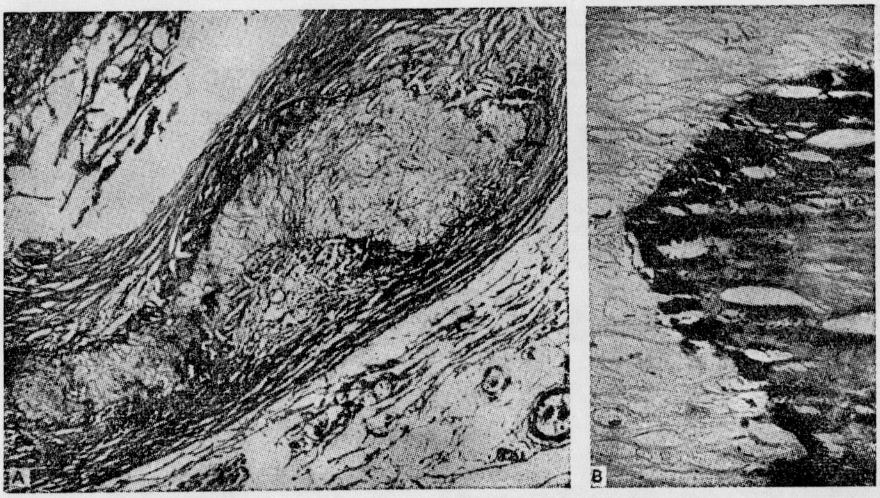

Figure 11. Varying degree of calcification in the necrotic areas of a vessel wall.

A, a necrotic sclerosed area in the wall of coronary artery; the peripheral portion shows early signs of calcification. Masson stain. Magnification 42 ×; *B*, substantial calcification of a necrotic area in the coronary artery wall. Stained with hematoxylin-eosin. Magnification 42 ×.

lesions occupies 50% or more of the intimal surface of the vessel) in persons dying from complications of atherosclerosis (Table 12). Here the maximum differences between the groups in the frequency of severe degrees of atherosclerosis are noted in the fifth and sixth decades of life. In subsequent decades these differences diminished somewhat: in patients dying from complications of atherosclerosis in the fifth and sixth decades of life severe degrees of atherosclerosis were four to five times as high. In the eighth decade of life the changes were only 1.5 times as frequent as in healthy subjects.

In subjects dying from complications of atherosclerosis the areas of vessel changes in atherosclerosis from the fifth to the eighth decade of life are less marked than in EHI. In healthy males the area with raised lesions in the abdominal aorta increases 3.2 times during this period and 4.5 times in females. In subjects dying from atherosclerosis the increases are 1.7 and 2.6, respectively. In the LAD coronary artery the area with raised lesions increases 2.4 times in healthy males and 4.5 times in females, but in subjects dying from atherosclerosis the increases are only 1.1 and 1.9 times.

The frequent presence of stenosis of the coronary arteries is a characteristic of the group dying from the complications of atherosclerosis. Stenosis of the coronary arteries by 50% or more of their lumen in this group is noted several times more frequently than in healthy subjects. The differences between the

Table 12. Prevalence of Severe Atherosclerosis in EHI (1) and Those Dying from Atherosclerosis (2)

Age in years	Subgroups	ThA		AA		LADCA		RCA	
		Males	Females	Males	Females	Males	Females	Males	Females
40–49	1	3.4	—	5.8	7.8	10.2	4.1	10.0	5.2
	2	9.1	—	30.3	5.3	47.2	22.2	40.9	22.3
50–59	1	8.0	6.3	22.7	16.9	16.0	9.9	18.2	8.8
	2	13.4	23.2	55.4	53.4	42.8	33.3	42.0	26.2
60–69	1	21.3	19.1	48.0	47.6	30.3	27.9	33.8	24.3
	2	33.8	32.0	69.2	65.3	65.8	51.8	62.0	50.5
70–79	1	25.4	32.1	55.0	60.3	42.3	42.0	40.4	39.2
	2	51.7	52.6	69.9	43.7	62.5	56.9	61.8	51.6

ThA, thoracic aorta; AA, abdominal aorta; LADCA, left anterior descending coronary artery; RCA, right coronary artery. Figures represent percent of cases with raised atherosclerotic changes in 50% or more of the intimal surface of a vessel.

groups were greater in the fifth and sixth decades of life (Table 13). This also indicates that in patients dying from complications of atherosclerosis, the process develops quite rapidly and quickly becomes serious.

Table 13. Prevalence of Stenosis of Coronary Arteries in EHI and in Subjects Dying from Atherosclerotic Complications without Hypertension

Groups	Age in years		
	40–49	50–59	60–69
Males			
Healthy	1.8 (324)*	8.5 (248)	14.6 (137)
Atherosclerosis	34.1 (44)	44.6 (139)	56.3 (222)
Females			
Healthy	0.9 (114)	4.1 (120)	16.5 (85)
Atherosclerosis	18.1 (11)	33.3 (27)	40.2 (144)

* Figures in brackets indicate number of observations. Other figures are the percentages of observations.

In the majority of cases with stenosis of the coronary arteries, atherosclerotic changes occupied more than 50% of the intimal surface of the artery, i.e., stenosis of the arteries develops in the setting of severe atherosclerosis; only occasionally was stenosis present as a result of one or two thick plaques, occupying only a small area of the vessel. Second, stenosis of the coronary arteries as a rule was noted in conjunction with calcification of these arteries. In 230 cases with stenosis of 50% or more of the lumen of the LAD coronary artery calcification was present in 90.9% cases. Only in 9.1% of the cases was stenosis of the artery not associated with calcification. Third, the prevalence of stenosis of the coronary arteries and the area with calcification in these arteries are directly proportional. In the LAD coronary artery, when the total area with atherosclerotic changes is more than 50% of the intimal surface, the frequency of stenosis related to the area with calcification was as follows: in the absence of calcification, stenosis of the artery was seen in 6.8% of the cases; when the area with calcification was 1 to 5% of the intimal surface, stenosis was noticed in 42.6%; and when the area with calcification occupied more than 10% of the intimal surface, stenosis was noticed in 81.1% of cases.

CONCLUSIONS

The data presented above show that atherosclerosis in healthy people and in subjects dying from complications of atherosclerosis develops progressively, but the atherosclerotic process is always more severe in the latter group.

Vessels with fatty streaks and/or fibrous plaques were noted more frequently in EHI; in subjects dying from atherosclerosis the prevalence of vessels with complicated lesions and calcifications was more marked. Raised lesions (fibrous plaques, complicated lesions, and calcification) in the aorta and coronary arteries in the group of subjects dying from complications of atherosclerosis always occupied a greater area of the intimal surface than in healthy people. But in EHI the extent of the area with lipidosis was considerably greater in the vessels studied. The variations in the ratio between the area with lipidosis and raised lesions in the vessels studied were probably due to development of fibrous plaques on the site of fatty streaks in subjects dying from complications of atherosclerosis.

Attention is drawn to the fact that the differences between the groups in the prevalence and degree of calcification in the aorta and coronary arteries diminish considerably with increasing age. In the eighth decade of life differences in calcification between the groups almost disappeared, although differences in the areas with fibrous plaques and complicated lesions persisted. These data show the importance not only of previous atherosclerotic changes but also of age and other factors in the development of calcification.

In subjects dying from complications of atherosclerosis, although development of atherosclerosis was accelerated with age, the differences in the degree of change between the fifth and eighth decades of life were less than in healthy people. This indicates that complications develop from atherosclerosis only when the atherosclerotic process has reached a certain stage.

3

Atherosclerosis and Diabetes Mellitus

Advances in the treatment of diabetes have led to a considerable increase in the life span of patients with this disorder. At the beginning of the twentieth century the average life span of a diabetic was 44.5 years, and by 1956–57 it was 64.7 years (Joslin, 1961). Mikhailenko (1959) found the average life span to be 60.5 years; the average age of diabetic patients who died from a cardiovascular disease was even greater, 66.4 years. In the 487 autopsies that we conducted in patients dying from diabetes mellitus, 87.3% of the subjects were 50 years or older.

With the rise in the average life span of patients with diabetes mellitus and the increase in the duration of the disease, the cause of death of these patients has changed considerably. Before the advent of insulin most patients with diabetes died from coma, tuberculosis or other infections, and only a few from cardiovascular diseases. Today the principal cause of death of patients suffering from diabetes mellitus, particularly those over the age of 50, is cardiovascular disease. Joslin *et al.* (1959) presented the data showing the cause of death in 18,055 patients with diabetes mellitus for a period of 60 years: in the years 1898–1912, 64% of patients died from a diabetic coma; 8.3% in 1922–34; 1% in 1956–57. Deaths from cardiovascular diseases were 17.5%, 54.4%, and 77.7%, respectively. However, we must note that there are considerable differences in the cause of death of young and old patients with diabetes mellitus. According to our data the cause of death of diabetic patients 50 years old or more is cardiovascular disease in approximately 70% of cases. In subjects below 50 years of age cardiovascular diseases account for only 14% of the deaths. As in earlier times, the main causes of death of young diabetics are coma or infectious diseases. In the last two decades diabetic glomerulosclerosis has often been found to be the cause of death in young patients with diabetes mellitus (Root and White, 1956). But according to our data, although the prevalence of diabetic glomerulosclerosis was high in young patients with diabetes, this complication of diabetes was rarely registered at the time of autopsy in either group above or below 50 years of age (in 5.3% and 1.2% of cases, respectively).

In diabetic patients atherosclerotic diseases of the heart (myocardial infarction, postinfarction cardiosclerosis) and blood vessels are frequently found. According to Clawson and Bell (1949), in male patients over 40 years of age, death due to coronary atherosclerosis was twice as frequent as in non-diabetics. For females the difference was threefold (in males 19.5% and 10.0%, and in females 17.4% and 5.8% of the cases, respectively). Analogous data have been presented by Thomas *et al.* (1956). However, the relationship between the development of atherosclerotic diseases (mainly myocardial infarction) and diabetes mellitus has not yet been settled. A number of workers (Sachsse, 1957; Della and Salda, 1966; Myasnikova, 1969) found a direct relationship between the prevalence of myocardial infarction in diabetic patients on the one hand and the severity and duration of diabetes on the other. But other workers (Liebow *et al.*, 1955; Moskovich, 1958; Ionash and Kozak, 1963) found no definite relationship between these two diseases. Ionash and Kozak (1963) found only a mild or moderate disorder of carbohydrate metabolism in the majority of diabetic patients with myocardial infarction. This disorder was often observed soon before the diagnosis of myocardial infarction, or the diabetes was noted only during hospitalization of the patient. The study of Büchele (1962) is also interesting. He noted latent disorders of carbohydrate metabolism in 42% of patients with myocardial infarction. Büchele believes that since no therapeutic measures had been taken to correct such latent disorders their significance in the development of cardiovascular diseases may be even greater than the overt types of diabetes which are treated.

Many authors noted sex variations in the prevalence of myocardial infarction, emphasizing the greater prevalence in males. The ratio between males and females among those dying from coronary disease, according to the data of Clawson and Bell (1949) is 5:3 and according to Ionash and Kozak (1963) 4:1. Among the diabetic patients the prevalence of myocardial infarction in both males and females was found to be more or less the same (Nathanson, 1932; Clawson and Bell, 1949; Feldman and Feldman, 1954; Czerkawsky, 1963; Ionash and Kozak, 1966). Analysis of our data showed that in patients with diabetes and without diabetes the myocardial lesions (myocardial infarction, cardiosclerosis) and stenosis of the coronary arteries were more frequent in males than in females, although the variations in sex in the diabetic group were less significant than those found by the above authors. In non-diabetics myocardial lesions in the age range of 50 to 59 years were present at a ratio of 2.6:1.0 in males and females; in the age range 60 to 69 years, 1.7:1.0; in the diabetic patients, 1.6:1.0 and 1.3:1.0, respectively.

The significance of atherosclerosis of the coronary arteries in the development of myocardial infarction in patients with diabetes has been discussed in the literature for many years. The more frequent development of myocardial infarction and coronary disease in diabetic patients is usually explained by the presence of severe atherosclerosis of the coronary arteries in these cases. However, it must be noted that the degree of atherosclerosis of the coronary arteries in myocardial infarction may be highly variable (Smol'yannikov and Naddachina, 1967; Vikhert and Matova, 1967; Sternby, 1968). Some workers (Smol'yannikov and Naddachina, 1967) have indicated that there are some clinico-anatomical peculiarities in the cardiac lesions in diabetes mellitus and have proposed that necrosis of the cardiac muscle is important in these cases. Often there is a trophic disorder rather than coronary insufficiency. The uncertainty and contradictions in the data presented once again indicate that it is very difficult to study the atherosclerotic process simply on the basis of clinical data. Only in recent years has coronary angiography been used extensively in living subjects, giving an opportunity to characterize objectively the status of coronary arteries in various pathological conditions of the heart. In particular these studies demonstrated that in cases of typical angina pectoris and clinically distinct cases of infarction there are nearly always (in 99% of cases) changes in the coronary arteries, mostly stenosis of these arteries (Proudfit and Shirey, 1966; Eliasch *et al.*, 1967). But we have seen no data on coronary angiography related to subjects suffering from diabetes mellitus. Therefore the study of this problem based on pathological data and comparison of the data obtained from control groups of EHI and from the groups of people dying from complications of atherosclerosis but not suffering from diabetes has added importance.

In addition to myocardial infarction, gangrene of the lower extremities often develops in diabetic patients. According to Bell (1950) gangrene of the legs is found 40 times more often in these patients than in other patients; he showed that the duration of diabetes had a significant effect in such cases. Goodman and colleagues (1950) noted occlusive disease in the lower extremities in 41 of 89 patients with diabetes mellitus, i.e., in almost half of the cases. Gangrene of the lower extremities is also found more frequently in those suffering from diabetes than in other patients, but the differences we observed between the groups are not so great. In diabetic patients between 50 and 79 years of age gangrene of the lower extremities was noted in 27.9% of the males and in 23.3% of the females; in the nondiabetics dying from the various complications of atherosclerosis, the rates were 7.8% and 4.8%, respectively. In the diabetic patients gangrene of the extremities was found four to five times more often than in nondiabetic subjects dying from the complications of atherosclerosis.

It is probable our data reflect the true incidence since they are based on extensive, randomly selected, uncomplicated cases of diabetes and atherosclerosis. It must be noted that the development of gangrene of the lower extremities is not necessarily a result of disease of the major vessels; it may also result from lesions of the small arteries, arterioles, capillaries, or venules (Klemashev, 1964; Funk, 1965; Blumenthal, 1968). Abramova (1967) demonstrated that disorders of the circulation in the lower extremities in patients with atherosclerosis without diabetes mellitus are due to major lesions of the large arteries. The atherosclerotic processes are localized mainly in the proximal parts of the arteries. On the contrary, in diabetic patients disorders of peripheral circulation are not only from atherosclerosis, but also from diabetic arteriosclerosis. The arteriosclerosis of the arteries of the lower extremities in diabetic patients is more pronounced in the arteries of the lower leg than those of the thigh. In all cases atherosclerotic plaques in diabetic patients are distributed in the distal parts of the large arteries of the leg, like the arteries of the foot and the intramuscular branches.

Haimovici (1961) and Klemashev (1964) likewise showed that in diabetes the atherosclerotic lesions are more extensive in nature, and that lesions are seen more frequently in the moderate-sized arteries of the leg and foot than in cases of atherosclerosis without associated diabetes.

It may be concluded that the development of gangrene of the lower extremities in diabetics results not only from atherosclerosis of the large vessels, but also from lesions of the smaller vessels.

Thus vascular changes are more frequent in diabetic patients over 50 years of age. Both atherosclerosis of the large arteries and aorta and diabetic arteriosclerosis are often present. The changes in the small vessels, particularly in the retina and kidneys, are specific for diabetes, according to many authors. These changes are usually dependent on the duration of the diabetes (Bell, 1952; Root and White, 1956; Kogan *et al.*, 1960; Madjari, 1961; Abramova, 1967; Robertson and Strong, 1968).

The atherosclerotic process in the vessels of patients with diabetes mellitus is not accompanied by any specific macroscopic signs. Comparison of groups of individuals with and without diabetes mellitus indicates that diabetics differ in the degree and severity of atherosclerosis but not in its qualitative characteristics. Numerous investigators have found that patients with diabetes mellitus have more severe atherosclerosis than other patients (Anichkov, 1935; LeCompte, 1945; Mitchell and Schwartz, 1965; Sternby, 1968). According to Hempel (1957) the atheromatous type of atherosclerosis is typical for diabetes mellitus, which is more severe and progressive in nature. It is true that some biochemical and histochemical studies apparently show several qualitative peculiarities in the atherosclerotic process in patients suffering from diabetes mellitus. A biochemical examination of the coronary vessels (Lundback and Peterson, 1953) revealed that in diabetic patients there is a decreased level of calcium and lecithin in the arteries and a twofold rise in the level of cephalin; the cholesterol and total phospholipid levels in the coronary arteries were the same in patients with diabetes and in subjects without diabetes. Similarly, the histochemical studies by Randerath and Diezel (1959) revealed some differences. They found that the levels of cholesterol esters and phospholipids were considerably higher in the old aortic plaques of diabetic patients than in the atherosclerotic plaques of nondiabetic subjects. In the nondiabetics the plaques contained more neutral lipids. In the opinion of these authors, a greater concentration of highly polymerized acid mucopolysaccharides is found in the plaques in patients with diabetic mellitus (mucopolysaccharide plaques). In our opinion the above differences are not fundamental in nature. They are simply signs of the progressive development of atherosclerosis in diabetes. In addition, the findings of Lundback and Peterson contradict the results of Randerath and Diezel. We give more credence to the information given by the former authors because they used more sophisticated methods of investigation.

The data showing that patients with diabetes mellitus generally die from cardiovascular diseases and the frequent detection of advanced atherosclerosis in diabetics have led many investigators to believe that diabetes hastens the development of atherosclerosis (Anichkov, 1935; Liebow and Hellerstein, 1949; Buschmann *et al.*, 1958; Joslin *et al.*, 1959; Myasnikov, 1960, 1965; Hodler, 1963; Tsyukhno, 1964; Myasnikov and Klemashev, 1965). This assumption is supported by the fact that the disorders of lipids, lipoproteins and glycoproteins in atherosclerosis and in diabetes mellitus are of the same nature (Myasnikov, 1960, 1965; Siperstein, 1964; Leites, 1967).

Others think that the frequent combination of atherosclerosis and diabetes is due to the development of diabetes secondary to atherosclerotic lesions in the vessels of the pancreas, and that the diabetes itself has no significant effect on the development of atherosclerosis (Naunyn, 1906; Moschkowitz, 1951; Boas, 1952; Moskovich, 1958; Vengerko, 1958; Liberman, 1965; Cooper *et al.*, 1960; Ionash and Kozak, 1963; Gruzina *et al.*, 1974).

Some facts to a certain extent support the above view.

First, diabetes mellitus markedly increases after 50 years of age when marked atherosclerotic changes also usually appear (Kogan-Yasnyi, 1957; Buschmann *et al.*, 1958; Egorova and Mezentsev, 1962; Genes, 1963; Pietschmann and Reinhardt, 1963).

Second, although many authors have noted the frequent combination of atherosclerosis and diabetes mellitus, they have failed to demonstrate a direct relationship between the severity and duration of diabetes and the degree of atherosclerosis and the frequency of myocardial infarction (Hart and Lisa, 1944; Naide, 1945; Tsukershtein, 1947; Boas, 1952; Schubert *et al.*, 1956, Mohnike, 1957; Moskovich, 1958; Ionash and Kozak, 1966). White and Wascow (1948) noted that the duration of diabetes is of greater importance in the development of atherosclerosis in the young than in the elderly.

Third, in the elderly the clinical signs of atherosclerosis often precede the development of diabetes mellitus (Moschkowitz, 1951; Yudanova and Solodun, 1964; Lautsevichus *et al.*, 1973).

Fourth, in atherosclerosis, particularly when essential hypertension is also present, changes are noticed in the vessels supplying the pancreas and the Islets of Langerhans that may lead to insulin deficiency (Boiko, 1957; Zhukov, 1959; Stepanov, 1966; Shvarts, 1967; Schubert *et al.*, 1956). This has been clearly demonstrated by Butkus (1967). He observed that fibrosis and lipomatosis of the pancreas and, similarly, changes in the Islets of Langerhans depended mainly on the degree of atherosclerosis in the splenic artery and the involvement of the sites of the splenic artery from which the arteries to the pancreas originate.

Fifth, in subjects suffering from atherosclerosis there are often disorders of carbohydrate metabolism, detected by carbohydrate tolerance tests (Kogan, 1936; Azerad *et al.*, 1963; Yudanova and Solodun, 1964; Liberman, 1965; Bahl, 1970).

It must also be noted that the combination of severe atherosclerosis and diabetes mellitus in isolated cases may be due to the presence of hypertension in diabetic patients (Lundback and Peterson, 1963; Myasnikov and Klemashev, 1965; Zaschoch, 1967; Fomenko and Tirkina, 1971), which according to most authors is seen in more than 50% of the patients with diabetes mellitus.

It has been established that both secondary and essential hypertension hasten the development of atherosclerotic changes (see chapter 10). This fact should be considered when conducting comparative studies of the degree of atherosclerosis of patients with diabetes mellitus as well as in studies of control groups.

Faber and Lund (1951) concluded that diabetes does not affect the development of atherosclerosis, but at the same time stressed that age and arterial pressure are the factors that determine the development of the disease.

Several investigators think that diabetes mellitus and atherosclerosis do not affect each other but develop simultaneously. The frequent combination of these disorders is probably due to genetic factors (Hart and Lisa, 1944; Boas, 1952; Liberman, 1965). In the opinion of Hart and Lisa individuals who are particularly resistant to atherosclerosis are also resistant to diabetes. According to several authors (Tsukershtein, 1947; Liberman, 1965; Davidenkova, 1970) not all forms of diabetes mellitus are genetically identical. This fact should also be kept in mind. Severe juvenile diabetes in all probability is a recessive hereditary disease, and the milder form of diabetes, which develops in mature and elderly people, has a dominant inheritance pattern. Genealogical, clinical, and biochemical investigations conducted by Liberman (1965) showed peculiar relationships between diabetes and atherosclerosis in various age groups. In the families of patients with juvenile diabetes she failed to find any increased predisposition to lipid disorders or atherosclerosis. On the contrary, in elderly diabetic patients the hereditary predisposition to a disorder of lipid metabolism and atherosclerosis was pronounced. The same was noted in patients with atherosclerosis.

This information is in agreement with the findings of others who showed that in young people diabetes is not usually associated with severe atherosclerosis (Naunyn, 1906; Hart and Lisa, 1944; Vengerko, 1958; Gruzina *et al.*, 1974).

The studies presented demonstrate that the interrelationship between diabetes mellitus and atherosclerosis remains unclear. A large number of clinical, biochemical, and pathological studies devoted to the problem are contradictory. Experimental studies in animals with alloxan-induced diabetes have also failed to clarify the issue.

According to Fischer (1961), Vadachkoriya (1964), Duff *et al.* (1954), and Still *et al.* (1964), alloxan diabetes retards the development of atherosclerosis, which develops following the administration of cholesterol. To many people who contended that diabetes accelerates atherosclerosis, these experimental results were unexpected. According to Duff and Payne (1950) this action is probably connected with an increase in the level of phospholipids and a decrease in the ratio of cholesterol to phospholipids in the blood in the case of alloxan diabetes. Jones *et al.* (1951) noted that in alloxan diabetes there is a rise in the SF40-100 fraction of lipoproteins and not in the SF10-30 fraction. They believe that the development of atherosclerosis stems not only from a high blood cholesterol level but also from complex protein and lipid disorders with the formation of SF10-30 types of lipoproteins.

According to Leites (1967) the behavior of lipolytic enzymes is different in various stages of alloxan diabetes. In the early stages of alloxan diabetes there is increased activity of lipolytic enzymes in most organs and in the aorta. On the other hand, in the late stages there is exhaustion of this adaptive mechanism, and the activity of lipolytic enzymes begins to fall in a number of organs and tissues, including those in the aorta. This is associated with a local rise in the level of lipids. Leites, although he noted certain changes in the activity of lipolytic enzymes in various organs and the aorta, unfortunately does not give the comparative characteristics of the degree of atherosclerosis in experimental animals with and without alloxan diabetes. In particular he has not shown whether there is any variation in the degree of atherosclerosis in the last stage of alloxan diabetes with the respective control groups, which might hold some interest for solving the problem of the interrelation between atherosclerosis and diabetes.

A review of all the statements regarding the interrelationship of atherosclerosis and diabetes mellitus reveals a major discrepancy of opinions. Frequent presence of atherosclerotic changes in the aorta and arteries in patients with diabetes mellitus is explained by different authors in different ways. The divergent views may be presented as follows: (1) diabetes mellitus leads to accelerated development of atherosclerotic changes; (2) existing pronounced atherosclerosis leads to or favors the development of diabetes mellitus; (3) diabetes mellitus and atherosclerosis, although they do not affect each other, develop simultaneously, having some prerequisites in common.

The contradictions regarding the interrelationship of diabetes mellitus and atherosclerosis primarily reflect the difficulty of analyzing the data. For the analysis of atherosclerosis certain groups of people should be selected who differ in only one symptom. Patients with diabetes mellitus often have other chronic diseases, and these may affect the development of atherosclerosis. Hence we have excluded cases with a combination of diabetes with other diseases (rheumatism, pulmonary tuberculosis, chronic pneumonia, malignant tumors) from the analysis or examined them separately (for example, the combination of diabetes with essential hypertension). For the above analysis 285 uncomplicated cases of diabetes mellitus not associated with any other chronic disease were selected (Table 14).

Table 14. Age and Sex Distribution of Diabetes Mellitus Cases

Age in years	10–19	20–29	30–39	40–49	50–59	60–69	70–79	Total
Male	1	2	5	10	27	33	26	104
Female	2	5	8	7	27	66	66	181
Total	3	7	13	17	54	99	92	285

In the groups of patients with diabetes 50 years of age and above, the cause of death differed considerably. The main causes of death in patients with diabetes mellitus who died prior to 50 years of age (38 of 40) were diabetic coma and various infections, often a combination of both. In this age group only two patients died from a cardiovascular disorder; gangrene of the lower extremities occurred in a 40-year-old female and myocardial infarction in a 48-year-old male. According to an investigation sponsored by WHO, myocardial infarction among males under 50 years of age, who died from various diseases, was found in 6% of cases (Vikhert, 1973).

In the older age groups (over 50 years of age) the cause of death of patients with diabetes was most frequently a cardiovascular disorder, 72% in males and 70.4% in females. On the other hand, infections leading to death (abscesses, inflammations, suppurative pyelonephritis, sepsis, etc.) were present in only 15.6% of the males and 17.7% the females. Diabetic coma as the cause of death (often in combination with infectious and vascular complications) occurred in 6.6% of the males and 11.4% of the females.

In males dying from the complications of atherosclerosis in combination with diabetes mellitus, myocardial infarction and postinfarction cardiosclerosis were present more frequently than in subjects dying from the complications of atherosclerosis without diabetes (66.7% and 55.7%, respectively, $p = 0.05$); the differences were less significant in the corresponding groups of females (46.4% versus 41.4% of the cases). The various types of cerebrovascular disorders in males suffering from diabetes occurred more frequently (30%) than in subjects dying from the complications of atherosclerosis without diabetes (18%); the differences between the corresponding groups of females were not significant (27.7% and 21.4%, respectively).

As already stated, gangrene of the lower extremities was present more frequently in diabetic patients (more than 35% of all cases) than in subjects dying from atherosclerosis without diabetes (less than 8% of cases). It is interesting that in diabetic patients there were simultaneous circulatory disorders in various organs; myocardial infarction with postinfarction cardiosclerosis and gangrene of the lower extremities were frequently noted.

Since the number of cases in the age groups up to 50 years was not high the mean values of the atherosclerotic process were calculated only for the age groups 30–39 and 40–49 years. In addition, each individual case of diabetes mellitus of this group was compared with the values characterizing the control group of EHI. For this purpose the standard deviation of the different parameters from the arithmetic mean of the control group was taken into account. If the value of these parameters in individual cases at the time of comparison with the corresponding values of a control group was more than double its standard deviation, the differences were considered statistically significant, i.e., $p \leqslant 0.05$ (Bailey, 1959; Plokhinskii, 1961).

On the whole the age-related changes of the different types of atherosclerosis followed the same pattern as was noted in the group of EHI (see chapter 1). The area with lipidosis in the aorta gradually increased with age and was maximal in the fourth decade of life in males (in the abdominal aorta, 21.4% of the intimal surface) and in females in the fifth decade of life (22.6%).

In older patients the area with lipidosis in the aorta gradually decreased, and by the eighth decade of life occupied only 3–4% of the intimal surface.

The area with fibrous plaques in the aorta in patients with diabetes mellitus gradually increased with age and was maximal in the seventh decade of life in males (thoracic aorta, 38.6 ± 3.5%, and abdominal aorta, 49.4 ± 3.5% of the intimal surface), and in the eighth decade of life in females (thoracic aorta, 48.2 ± 2.0%, abdominal aorta, 50.1 ± 1.9%).

In the aorta complicated lesions and calcification were present in diabetic patients in the fourth and fifth decades of life. In the aorta in males, complicated lesions often occupied a considerably greater area than in females; in the eighth decade of life in the thoracic aorta the area with such lesions in males was 6.5 ± 2.0% and in the abdominal aorta, 11.4 ± 2.7% of the intimal surface; in females it was 2.8 ± 0.4% and 6.1 ± 1.4%, respectively. The differences in calcification of the aorta were less significant. Usually in subjects up to 70 years of age the area with calcification in the aorta was somewhat greater in males, but by the eighth decade of life the relationship was reversed (7.6 ± 2.5% of the intimal surface in the abdominal aorta of males and 13.7 ± 1.8% in females).

In the coronary arteries the general features of the development of atherosclerosis in diabetics followed the same pattern as in the group of healthy people and those dying from atherosclerosis. In the coronary arteries the area with lipidosis in diabetic patients belonging to all the age groups was not as high as in the aorta, and usually occupied less than 2 to 5% of the intimal surface of a vessel. The area with fibrous plaques in the coronary arteries gradually increased with age and was maximal in the seventh or eighth decade of life, occupying about 50% of the intimal surface. In the coronary arteries complicated lesions were present in patients with diabetes over 40 years of age. The average area of these lesions was usually not more than 1% of the intimal surface. In patients with diabetes calcification of the coronary arteries was present from the fourth decade in males and from the fifth decade in females. The area with calcification gradually increased with age and was maximal in subjects over 70 years of age, occupying 10–15% of the area of the vessel.

The extent of all types of atherosclerotic changes was maximal in the LAD coronary artery; the changes were almost of the same degree in the right coronary artery and the left circumflex coronary artery.

An analysis showing the ratio of various types of atherosclerotic changes demonstrates that in subjects under 50 years of age the total area with changes in both parts of the aorta was primarily due to fatty streaks; in subjects over 50 years of age fibrous plaques were the primary finding. In subjects over 40 years of age fibrous plaques are the main type of change in the coronary arteries (i.e., occupy the maximal area).

Attention is drawn to the fact that in both parts of the aorta atherosclerotic changes in males and in females suffering from diabetes were either uniform in both groups or were more frequent in females; in the coronary arteries, as a rule, the changes were more pronounced in males than in females.

In diabetes stenosis of the coronary arteries (narrowing of the lumen by 50% or more) was found from the fifth decade of life in males and from the sixth in females. In the age range between 50 and 79 stenoses were present in 41.1% of cases in males and 37.9% in females.

We offer a comparative analysis of the degree of atherosclerotic changes in patients with diabetes mellitus, in EHI and in those dying from the complications of atherosclerosis.

In the age group between 10 and 19 years, there were only three cases (the duration of diabetes was not more than a year). In all the cases only fatty streaks in both parts of the aorta were noted; the other types of atherosclerotic changes were absent. In the coronary arteries, too, there were only fatty streaks in two cases and in one case no change was seen. The extent of fatty streaks was the same as in the control groups of EHI.

In the age group between 20 and 29 years there were seven cases (two males and five females). The duration of the disease varied from one month to 17 years. In five cases the atherosclerotic changes were extensive; as a rule, these changes were noted in one or two vessels, but not in all five of the vessels studied. Altogether 33 vessels were studied in this age group; in only 10 were the atherosclerotic changes more marked than the average values observed in a group of healthy people. In three vessels the major finding was an area with lipidosis, in seven, an area with fibrous plaques; the duration of diabetes in these cases was for 9, 11, and 17 years. Neither complicated lesions nor calcification of the vessels were noted.

In the age group 30 to 39 years there were 13 cases (five males and eight females); 65 vessels were studied. The extent of atherosclerotic changes was considerably greater than normal in only nine vessels belonging to six patients with diabetes; the remaining vessels were the same as in a control group of healthy people. In the six cases the duration of diabetes was 2, 3, 3–4, 4–5, and 8 years. In the remaining cases, where the extent of atherosclerotic changes was the same as in the control group, the duration of diabetes varied from six months to 10 years.

In the age group 40 to 49 years there were 17 cases (ten males and seven females); 82 aortas and coronary arteries were studied in this age group. In only nine vessels was the extent of atherosclerotic change greater than in the control groups; in the remaining vessels these changes were within the normal limits of a control group of healthy people. In five out of nine vessels the abnormal area was occupied by fibrous plaques, and in four it was occupied by fatty streaks. In these nine vessels belonging to six cases the atherosclerotic changes were more extensive in four cases in one vessel only, in two vessels in one case, and in three vessels in three cases. The duration of diabetes in these cases was respectively 1, 9, and 10 years, and in one case diabetes was first detected at the last hospitalization. In two cases the duration of diabetes could not be ascertained. In the remaining 11 cases the duration of diabetes varied from six months to 13 years.

The data on 40 cases with diabetes mellitus in subjects up to 50 years of age demonstrate that the extent of atherosclerotic changes in the vessels studied was very rarely significantly greater than the corresponding control groups of healthy people. Often the extent of fibrous plaques (Fig. 12) and fatty streaks was essentially the same or even lower than in the control groups. Altogether 191 vessels (usually two segments of aorta and three coronary arteries in each case) were studied in the age groups up to 50 years. The area with fibrous plaques in 21 vessels (10.9%) and the area with lipidosis in only 9 vessels (4.7%) was significantly greater compared with a control group of healthy people.

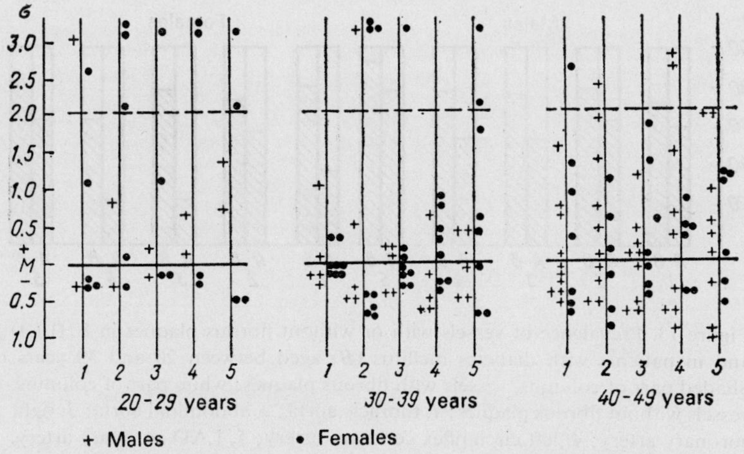

Figure 12. Area occupied by fibrous plaques in vessels of patients with diabetes mellitus as compared with that of EHI (control group). Ordinate shows deviation σ; *M*, mean (arithmetic) of control groups; σ, standard deviations of control groups. *1*, thoracic aorta; *2*, abdominal aorta; *3*, right coronary artery; *4*, left circumflex coronary artery; *5*, LAD coronary artery.

It should be noted that the above comparisons were conducted with the mean values of a group of healthy subjects. Among them there were considerable variations in the degree of atherosclerosis both above and below the mean values. In the healthy group there were more individuals with more pronounced atherosclerosis than in the group of diabetic patients.

Thus the degree of atherosclerotic change in most of the vessels in the presence of diabetes was the same as in a control group of healthy people. However, in diabetes mellitus (particularly in the age group between 20 and 39 years) vessels with fibrous plaques were encountered more frequently than in EHI. The differences were maximal in females in respect to prevalence of fibrous plaques in the coronary vessels (Fig. 13). In subjects with diabetes in the age groups 30–39 and 40–49 years, the mean data showing the area with atherosclerotic changes in the vessels studied were calculated in a similar manner. The differences between the diabetic patients and the EHI in the degree of atherosclerosis, both in the aorta and in the coronary arteries, were not great and were not statistically significant; moreover, the changes were not of the same magnitude. More often, particularly in females, the changes were more extensive in patients suffering from diabetes mellitus; in 45 of 100 comparisons made between the groups the changes occupied a greater area in patients with diabetes mellitus; the changes were greater in the EHI in 36 comparisons and in the remaining comparisons no differences were found between the groups.

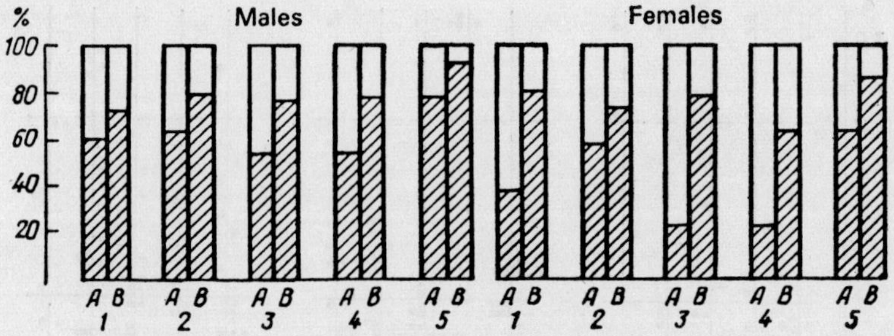

Figure 13. Prevalence of vessels with or without fibrous plaques in EHI (*A*) and in patients with diabetes mellitus (*B*) aged between 20 and 39 years. Shaded part of columns, vessels with fibrous plaques; white part of columns, vessels without fibrous plaques; *1*, thoracic aorta; *2*, abdominal aorta; *3*, right coronary artery; *4*, left circumflex coronary artery; *5*, LAD coronary artery.

Completely different results were obtained during an analysis of atherosclerotic changes in patients over age 50 with diabetes mellitus. In these patients the total area with atherosclerotic changes in all the vessels was larger than in a group of EHI. The observed increase in the total area of change in patients with diabetes mellitus was primarily due to raised lesions in the vessels (Table 15). When the areas with lipidosis in the vessels were compared the differences between the groups were not significant.

In the analysis of the components of raised lesions in the aorta and coronary arteries maximal differences were noted in relation to fibrous plaques (Table 15).

Comparison of the degree of atherosclerotic change in diabetic patients and in subjects dying from the various complications of atherosclerosis failed to reveal statistically significant differences. Among these groups there were no differences in the total area showing changes nor in the individual types of atherosclerosis, particularly complicated lesions and calcification. In subjects dying from the complications of atherosclerosis there was a tendency toward a higher degree of complicated lesions and calcification in the coronary arteries. The absence of significant differences between these groups in the degree of atherosclerotic changes in the aorta and coronary arteries is due to the greater prevalence of lethal complications of atherosclerosis in the group of patients with diabetes mellitus.

The degree of atherosclerotic changes in the vessels of those dying from the complications of atherosclerosis did not depend on its association with diabetes mellitus. Only in females with diabetes between 50 and 59 years of age did raised lesions (mainly fibrous plaques and calcification) occupy a significantly greater area compared with subjects dying from the complications of atherosclerosis without accompanying diabetes (Fig. 14). The prevalence of stenosis of the coronary arteries in the subjects dying from the complications

Table 15. Mean Area with Fibrous Plaques, Complicated Lesions, and Calcification in Vessels of EHI (1) and of Patients with Diabetes Mellitus (2)

Age in years	Groups	Thoracic aorta			Abdominal aorta			LAD coronary artery		
		FbPl	Co	Ca	FbPl	Co	Ca	FbPl	Co	Ca
Males										
50–59	1	14.4	0.3	0.2	25.8	1.4	1.5	27.0	0.0	2.4
	2	25.7*	1.0	0.5	41.0*	5.4*	3.0	44.2*	0.1	3.2
60–69	1	28.4	1.0	1.1	40.7	3.3	6.2	35.0	0.2	5.6
	2	38.6*	1.2	0.7	48.4*	5.9*	4.7	49.0*	0.9	6.1
70–79	1	33.6	2.0	2.0	39.7	2.9	7.2	38.9	0.5	10.8
	2	38.6	6.5*	1.5	41.2	11.4*	7.6	43.6	0.2	14.8
Age-standardized index	1	25.5*	1.1	1.1	35.4	2.5	4.9	33.9	0.3	6.3
	2	34.3*	2.9	0.9	43.5*	7.6*	5.1	45.6*	0.4	8.0
Females										
50–59	1	10.6	0.1	0.1	20.8	0.4	1.1	17.8	0.0	1.1
	2	30.8*	0.8*	1.4	40.7*	2.8*	6.9*	38.4*	0.0	2.7
60–69	1	26.5	0.5	1.1	36.5	1.3	3.9	27.5	0.1	5.3
	2	40.3*	1.3*	1.1	48.8*	4.4	6.0	45.5*	0.7	5.0
70–79	1	42.1	1.2	3.0	45.1	1.9	8.7	37.6	0.2	3.1
	2	48.2*	2.9*	3.4	50.1	6.1*	13.7*	41.9	0.1	8.5*
Age-standardized index	1	26.4	0.6	1.4	34.1	1.2	4.6	27.6	0.1	2.8
	2	39.8*	1.7*	2.0	46.5*	4.4*	8.9*	41.6*	0.3	5.4*

* Differences between the groups are statistically significant ($p \leqslant 0.05$). FbPl, fibrous plaques; Co, complicated lesions; Ca, calcification. Diseased areas given as percentage of intimal surface in vessels.

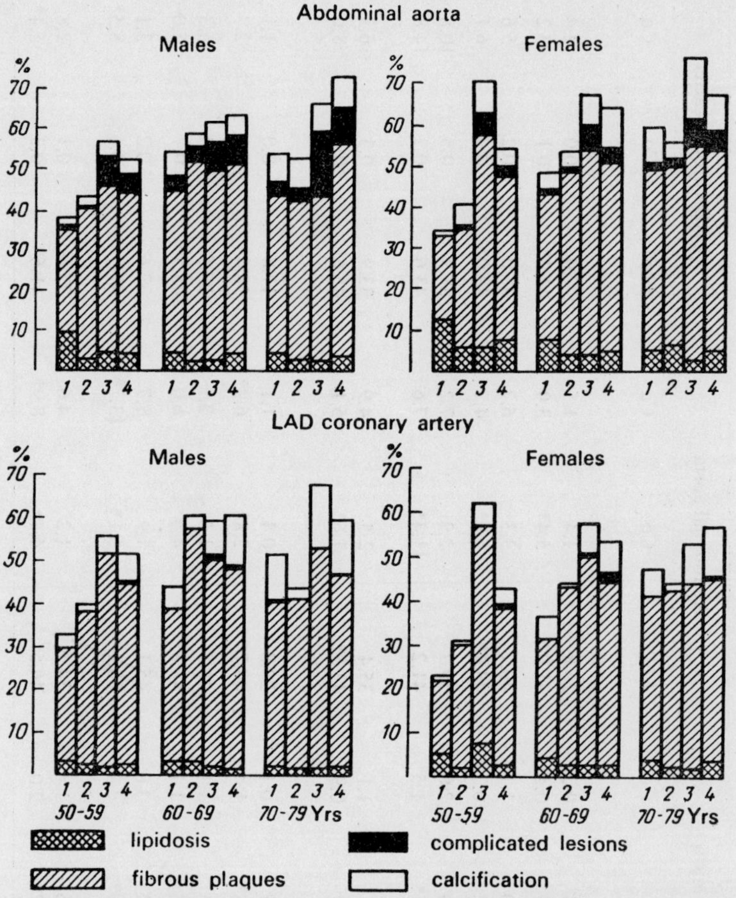

Figure 14. Area with atherosclerotic changes in abdominal aorta and LAD coronary artery. *1*, EHI; *2*, patients with diabetes mellitus; *3*, patients dying from complications of atherosclerosis accompanied by diabetes mellitus; *4*, patients dying from complications of atherosclerosis not accompanied by diabetes mellitus. Ordinate shows changes in intimal surface in percentages.

of atherosclerosis did not depend on the presence of diabetes mellitus. Stenosis of the coronary arteries by 50% or more of their lumen was found in males between 50 and 59 years dying from the complications of atherosclerosis accompanied by diabetes in 41.1% of cases and in 37.9% of the females. The figures were 42.3% and 39.5%, respectively, in cases not associated with diabetes.

We analyzed the extent and features of atherosclerosis in diabetic patients, depending on the cause of death. The cases were divided into two main subgroups. The first subgroup contained diabetic patients dying from the various complications of atherosclerosis; the second contained patients in which the cause of death was not related to atherosclerosis (34 males and 47 females). In the second subgroup, diabetic coma and various infectious diseases were the most frequent causes of death, but there were no signs of coronary, cerebral, or peripheral circulatory disorders. In this subgroup the atherosclerotic changes in the vessels were less pronounced than in subjects dying from the various complications of atherosclerosis both with and without associated diabetes. Maximal differences between comparable subgroups were noted in the extent of raised lesions: in the aorta complicated lesions, and to a lesser degree fibrous plaques and calcification, were more extensive; in the coronary arteries fibrous plaques were more extensive (Fig. 14).

In the diabetic patients in whom the cause of death was not related to atherosclerosis, the extent of atherosclerotic changes was somewhat greater than in EHI. The differences between the subgroups were statistically significant only in isolated comparisons. Moreover, these differences decreased with advancing age: in the ages between 50 and 59 years they were not great, between 60 and 69 years they were considerably reduced, and between 70 and 79 years the changes were even somewhat less in patients with diabetes mellitus who did not die from atherosclerosis (compared with EHI). Cases of diabetes mellitus associated with hypertension constitute a very large group. In the present work 128 such cases (45 males and 83 females between 50 and 79 years of age) have been analyzed.

The data presented in Table 16 show that the degree of atherosclerotic change in the vessels of diabetic patients with hypertension is greater than in

Table 16. Age-standardized (50–79 years) Indices of Areas with Raised Lesions in Diabetic and Hypertensive Patients

Groups	ThA	AA	RCA	LCCA	LADCA
Males					
1	38.3	56.2	48.8	46.8	54.1
2	48.2*	62.9*	58.4*	61.0*	69.5*
3	47.3*	66.0*	64.6*	60.3*	63.4*
Females					
1	43.3	59.8	44.7	41.5	48.0
2	60.0*	72.4*	55.6*	53.8*	65.1*
3	51.4*	69.9*	47.7	48.3*	52.0

ThA, thoracic aorta; AA, abdominal aorta; RCA, right coronary artery; LCCA, left circumflex coronary artery; LADCA, LAD coronary artery; 1, diabetes mellitus without hypertension; 2, diabetes mellitus with hypertension; 3, hypertension without diabetes mellitus.

* Statistically significant differences between 1 and remaining groups ($p \leqslant 0.05$). Diseased area given as a percentage of intimal surface of vessel.

patients with diabetes mellitus without hypertension (this analysis includes those who died from the complications of atherosclerosis). These data confirm the results of several workers who have shown that hypertension accelerates the development of atherosclerosis.

There are some notable features of atherosclerosis in the subjects with essential hypertension depending on the accompanying diabetes mellitus. In males suffering from essential hypertension the degree of atherosclerosis in the aorta and coronary arteries was practically the same in both subgroups (i.e., with or without diabetes); in females the severity of atherosclerosis was generally greater when combined with hypertension and diabetes mellitus (Table 16).

There was a tendency of patients with hypertension and diabetes to develop complicated lesions whose area was somewhat greater (especially in the aorta) than in EHI.

The data showing the absence of significant differences in the degree of atherosclerosis in males suffering from essential hypertension, depending on accompanying diabetes mellitus, mainly indicate the predominant role of hypertension in the development of atherosclerosis. The effect of diabetes mellitus on the development of atherosclerosis is noticeable in females suffering from hypertension.

In the absence of diabetes mellitus there are significant differences in the prevalence of coronary stenosis in subjects with hypertension and in subjects dying from the complications of atherosclerosis. With hypertension stenosis of the coronary arteries is found in 56.5% of the males in the sixth and seventh decades of life; in females, in 47% of cases; in subjects dying from the complications of atherosclerosis stenosis is present in 47.5% and 42.5% of the cases, respectively. In the presence of diabetes mellitus there were no differences between these groups in the prevalence of stenosis of the coronary arteries. It may be presumed from these data that diabetes mellitus does not favor the development of stenosis of the coronary arteries to a greater extent than hypertension.

The data allow us to draw several conclusions. First of all, differences in the degree of the atherosclerotic process between individual subgroups of patients with diabetes mellitus depended on the age of the patients and the cause of death and accompanying diseases, especially hypertension. Many comparisons that have been made of the degree of atherosclerosis in patients with diabetes mellitus and patients dying of other causes are inadequate, because of major differences in composition of the groups. These differences should be considered when comparative studies of the effect of diabetes mellitus on the development of atherosclerosis are conducted. The present work covers the degree of atherosclerosis in several groups of diabetics: (1) all cases of diabetes mellitus in the absence of accompanying diseases; (2) cases of diabetes mellitus where the cause of death of the patient was atherosclerosis; (3) cases of diabetes mellitus where the cause of death of the patient was not atherosclerosis; (4) cases of diabetes mellitus accompanied by hypertension. A comparison of the groups was done with a group of EHI, with a group dying from the complications of atherosclerosis, and with a group of people having hypertension without accompanying diabetes. Several authors have recently tried to perform differential comparisons (Mitchell and Schwartz, 1965; Sternby, 1968), which are more suitable for explaining the interrelationship between diabetes mellitus and atherosclerosis.

Atherosclerosis in patients with diabetes varied depending on age. Diabetics dying before 50 years of age (40 cases) showed more extensive atherosclerotic changes in isolated vessels in only 17 cases. In this age group (12–49 years) 191 vessels were studied. In only 21 vessels (11%) was the area with fibrous plaques significantly greater than in EHI, and in only 9 vessels (4.7%) was the area with lipidosis greater.

The duration of diabetes has a role in the development of atherosclerosis, although the relationship is not direct. In patients with diabetes for five years intense atherosclerosis in isolated vessels was more frequent than in subjects having diabetes for less than five years. However, in some cases there was no intensification of atherosclerosis even when the duration of diabetes was 10 to 13 years.

Our data do not indicate that diabetes has any significant accelerating effect on the development of atherosclerosis in subjects less than 50 years of age. Data revealing the cause of death of these patients support the above view. In most cases coma or acute infectious diseases were reported to be the cause of death; only two of 40 patients in this group died from cardiovascular disorders.

On the other hand, in diabetics over 50 years of age the prevalence of atherosclerotic changes in all the vessels studied was usually much more extensive than in healthy people. But they differed less from those who died from the various complications of atherosclerosis without diabetes. This occurs because the cause of death of those over 50 years of age suffering from diabetes was often connected with pathology of the cardiovascular system (72.3% in males and 70.4% in females).

The observations made by several investigators (Hart and Liza, 1944; Root and White, 1956; Vengerko, 1958; Genes, 1963) and our own observations indicate that in young patients diabetes rarely leads to the development of severe atherosclerosis. The characteristic courses of diabetes in different age groups have their own names: juvenile diabetes and maturity onset diabetes. These also differ from each other in their genetic features.

Comparison of atherosclerosis in subjects dying from various complications of atherosclerosis, with or without diabetes, revealed significant differences between these groups only in females between 50 and 59 years of age. In subsequent decades of life the differences between the groups were not significant, although in the females suffering from diabetes the atherosclerotic changes were often somewhat more marked. Mitchell and Schwartz (1965) also did not find significant differences in the degree of atherosclerosis in females with myocardial infarction, with or without diabetes. Data showing the prevalence of stenosis of the coronary arteries and the prevalence of myocardial infarction and post-infarction cardiosclerosis also show no significant differences between the groups of those who died from the complications of atherosclerosis, with or without diabetes mellitus.

In diabetic patients whose death was not caused by atherosclerosis the area with atherosclerotic changes in the sixth and seventh decades of life was greater as compared with that of healthy people, although the differences between these groups usually were not statistically significant.

According to our data a combination of diabetes mellitus and hypertension is associated with more rapid development of atherosclerosis. Moreover, the degree of atherosclerosis in males suffering from diabetes depends on the association of essential hypertension to a greater extent than in females.

Since diabetic subjects over 50 years of age show pronounced atherosclerotic changes both with and without hypertension, it is not possible to agree with the opinion of several authors (Faber and Lund, 1951; Robertson, 1962) that hypertension is the main cause of the accelerated development of atherosclerosis in diabetes. Others agree that hypertension is not necessary for the development of severe atherosclerosis in diabetes mellitus patients (Anichkov, 1947; Myasnikov, 1960, 1965; Sternby, 1968; Myasnikov Jr., 1969).

There are many reports that there is a higher frequency of myocardial infarction and atherosclerosis in subjects suffering from diabetes (Clawson and Bell, 1949; Feldman and Feldman, 1954; Myasnikov and Klemashev, 1965; Lubetzki, 1973). The data were obtained mainly from comparisons of groups of diabetic patients with groups of patients dying from all other causes. When compared with these groups, a greater frequency of myocardial infarction and a higher degree of atherosclerosis are noted in patients who had diabetes. Similarly, the composition of the group with respect to death due to atherosclerosis, hypertension, or malignant tumors differed from author to author. Since the number of persons dying from atherosclerosis and hypertension (without diabetes mellitus) increases with age, the differences in the degree of atherosclerotic changes between the above groups are not significant; moreover, in older age groups (above 70 years) the changes may even be somewhat more in nondiabetic subjects.

Thus the accelerated development of atherosclerosis in diabetes is not always caused by the diabetes. It can well be argued that often in people over 50 years of age diabetes appears in the presence of pronounced atherosclerosis, which may have led to the development of diabetes. Some facts support this view.

First, in patients under age 50 with diabetes the atherosclerotic changes are very rarely more pronounced than in EHI; in patients over 50 years of age the changes are usually as pronounced as changes in subjects dying from the various complications of atherosclerosis without diabetes. Second, diabetes rises sharply in individuals over 50 at the same time that pronounced atherosclerotic changes are also usually noted in the aorta and the arteries supplying the pancreas. Third, there is no direct relationship between the severity and duration of diabetes and the degree of atherosclerosis. Fourth, clinical treatment of diabetes mellitus is usually associated with normalization of the disorders of lipid metabolism.

The data supporting the possibility that the development of diabetes mellitus in subjects over 50 years of age is due to atherosclerosis do not exclude the possibility that diabetes mellitus accelerates atherosclerosis. To a certain degree the data comparing the degree of atherosclerosis in the aorta and coronary arteries of diabetic patients dying mainly from infectious diseases and coma with EHI can be cited in support of the above. The atherosclerotic process in the former group is usually more advanced than in healthy subjects. However, in most of the comparisons the differences between these groups in the area with atherosclerotic changes were not significant. This means that only a tendency to accelerated development of atherosclerosis in the presence of diabetes may be present. The data showing more severe atherosclerosis in those between 50 and 59 years of age with complications of atherosclerosis in combination with diabetes mellitus than in those without such a combination have the same implication. Despite this, it appears to us that the effect of diabetes mellitus on the development of atherosclerosis is probably not so important as has been suggested by many researchers.

It should be noted that the study of the effect of diabetes on the development of atherosclerosis has numerous difficulties. These are particularly due to the great variations regarding the duration of the diabetes mellitus, the nature of the course of the disease (mild or severe diabetes), the regularity and effectiveness of treatment, the degree and distribution of specific changes in the small vessels, and the effect of accompanying diseases on the course of atherosclerosis.

4

Atherosclerosis and Malignant Tumors

The effect of malignant tumors on the development of atherosclerosis has attracted the attention of specialists for many years. At present malignant tumors and the various complications of atherosclerosis are the main causes of death in the older age groups. The two diseases are very commonly combined.

A combination of malignant tumors with atherosclerosis is probably more common than atherosclerosis observed in all other groups of the population. According to separate epidemiological data (Vanecek *et al.*, 1967) the degree of atherosclerosis in the aorta and coronary arteries in the residents of Ryazan was less pronounced than in the residents of Tallin, Malmö, and Prague. According to our data, in patients dying from malignant tumors in Ryazan atherosclerosis in the aorta and coronary arteries was less pronounced than in similar patients in Tallin. Gamiyants (1964), who studied atherosclerosis in Samarkand residents dying from malignant tumors, found that in the natives atherosclerotic lesions were half as common as in the immigrant population (5.7% and 12.5%, respectively). The author attributes this to the lower incidence of atherosclerosis among the native population.

To judge the prevalence and degree of atherosclerosis in patients with malignant tumors, researchers have in most cases relied on retrospective analysis of autopsy forms; very rarely have the vessels been studied directly (Leites, 1932; Anichkov, 1935; Schneider, 1936; Juhl, 1955, 1957; Parrish, 1961; Sementsov, 1962; Zav'yalova, 1965; Giertsen, 1966; Parrish *et al.*, 1966). Most researchers have found that the degree of atherosclerosis is less pronounced in patients dying of malignant tumors than in all other deaths; it is emphasized that severe degrees of atherosclerosis are rarely seen in malignant patients. Kadas (1961) noted mild atherosclerosis in 96.4% and moderate atherosclerosis in 3.3% of those dying from malignant tumors. In patients dying of all causes mild atherosclerosis was noted in only 26.1% and moderate or severe atherosclerosis in 73.2%. According to Grosse (1960) the differences in the degree of atherosclerosis in subjects with and without malignant tumors were most distinct in middle age and diminished in the older age groups.

The developmental characteristics of atherosclerosis in patients with malignant tumors, as in other diseases, are revealed by conducting comparative studies of atherosclerosis in various groups of people. It is presumed that the natural course of the atherosclerotic process can be traced first of all in EHI dying from accidental causes. This group of people was used to demonstrate the characteristics of the course of atherosclerosis in patients with malignant tumors (Juhl, 1957; Parrish, 1961). The results of a comparative study of atherosclerosis depend heavily upon the composition of the control group. Parrish (1961) compared the degree of atherosclerosis in patients dying from carcinoma in various locations with those dying from other diseases; he found less pronounced atherosclerosis in the patients with malignancy. However, when a group of patients with carcinoma was compared with a group of victims of accidental death, no differences were present. In the opinion of the author, the group of victims with accidental death is a more suitable control for the evaluation of the rate of development of atherosclerosis. The apparent differences in atherosclerosis between patients dying from carcinoma and those dying from all other causes result from special selection and do not reflect the true situation. Among those dying from all other causes there were patients who died from the complications of atherosclerosis and hypertension. Parrish came to the conclusion that in reality there is neither a positive nor a negative correlation between cancer and atherosclerosis. Giertsen (1966) holds a similar view. This is based on the biochemical characteristic of the severity of atherosclerosis in respect to the ratio of cholesterol to phospholipids. He noted a low degree of atherosclerosis in subjects dying from malignant tumors in comparison with all other patients. When arterial hypertension and atherosclerotic heart diseases were excluded from the control group the differences between the groups were less distinct and the differences in the degree of atherosclerosis in the major arteries of the brain disappeared completely.

Very little information is available with regard to the characteristics of individual types of atherosclerotic changes in malignant tumors. According to many authors lipidosis of the vessels (Kremnev, 1951; Juhl, 1955; Eilersen and Faber, 1960) is less pronounced in subjects dying from carcinoma than in other patients. Wilens (1947) noted smaller deposits of lipids only in subjects with a considerable loss of body weight; he found no decrease in the degree of other types of atherosclerotic change. Some investigators (Eakins, 1965), however, failed to note any significant differences in the degree of lipidosis of the vessels in subjects dying from carcinoma or other diseases.

Reports showing calcification of the arteries in malignant tumors are somewhat more numerous (Sedov, 1967; Vikhert *et al.*, 1970). According to the materials of Vikhert *et al.*, calcification of the arteries in patients with carcinoma in various locations (except lung cancer) was somewhat less in degree than in EHI. According to the radiologic data of Winkelstein *et al.* (1959), the prevalence of calcification of the thoracic and abdominal aortas was practically the same in patients with and without cancer. Sedov (1967) and Eakins (1965) found no differences in the degree of calcification in pathologic specimens from these groups of patients. On the contrary, during radiologic study of the abdominal aorta Elkeles (1963) in most cases noted extensive calcification in the presence of slowly developing carcinoma (duration of cancer up to 15 years). According to Elkeles (1953, 1956), Dungul and Benidiktsson (1958), and Fotopoulus *et al.* (1962), the frequency of calcification of the aorta was lowest in the case of gastric carcinoma. Elkeles contends that in peptic ulcer there is very often extensive calcification of the abdominal aorta, and this characteristic can serve as a differential sign between gastric carcinoma and the peptic ulcer.

According to Elkeles (1953, 1956) extensive calcification of the abdominal aorta is rarely observed not only in the presence of gastric carcinoma, but also in the presence of carcinoma of the breast and the prostate. In carcinomas of the respiratory organs the author noted calcification of the same frequency as in the control group. A number of authors emphasize that hypercalcemia resulting from the localization of a tumor in bone may be the cause of pronounced calcification of the arteries (Fanconi, 1960; Camus, 1963).

Since severe types of atherosclerosis are rarely observed in subjects dying from carcinoma, several authors consider that an antagonism exists between predispositions to the two diseases (Schneider, 1936; Wanscher, 1951; Juhl, 1955; Elkeles, 1956). According to some investigators genetic mechanisms (Elkeles, 1963) or constitutional factors (Tiedemann, 1957; Freudenberg, 1958) cause these predispositions. Little is known of genetic factors that might predispose to the development of one disease and at the same time inhibit the development of another, but this is very interesting for study.

Elkeles (1956) suggests that there are differences in the relations between atherosclerosis and various carcinomas. In carcinomas due to genetic or hormonal factors atherosclerosis with extensive calcification is rarely seen; in carcinomas that are produced primarily by exogenous carcinogenic agents the degree of atherosclerosis (and calcification) does not differ from that of the control groups. However, this view remains hypothetical and is not yet supported by data.

Several investigators believe that the disorders of lipids and other metabolic problems cause the low degree of atherosclerosis in patients with malignant tumors (Jowett, 1931; Medes *et al.*, 1953; Medvedeva, 1955). Tichy *et al.* (1953) suggest that metabolic disorders which appear with age predispose either to the development of atherosclerosis or to the appearance of carcinoma.

According to Juhl (1955) a malignant tumor inhibits the development of atherosclerosis, since cholesterol and its derivatives have some role in the development and growth of a carcinoma.

Jowett (1931) and Medes *et al.* (1953) noted that rapidly growing tumors contain more cholesterol and phospholipids than other tissues. In the opinion of Medes *et al.* (1953) most of the tumor cholesterol appears in the tumor not by local synthesis in the tumor but by absorption of cholesterol from the blood; the rapidly growing peripheral part of a tumor contains more cholesterol ester than the central parts, which are often necrotic. Moreover, malignant tumors contain more cholesterol than benign tumors. Despite a large number of studies the issue remains unclear. However, in all probability the hypocholesteremia often noted with malignant tumors is only partly due to absorption of blood cholesterol by the tumor. Other factors, for example, disorders of the liver and endocrine glands, may also have an important role in the lipid metabolism of patients with malignant neoplasms.

We studied the degree of atherosclerotic changes in malignant tumors in the different decades of life for all types of malignant tumors and separately for some types of carcinomas. Cases where a combination of malignant tumors with atherosclerosis had been noted, regardless of whether atherosclerosis was diagnosed as the main or as an accompanying disease, were included in the investigation. Altogether 1,803 cases with malignant tumors (876 males and 927 females, 30–79 years of age) were studied; each decade of life comprised more than 200 cases except the fourth, in which there were 123 cases (63 males and 60 females).

In subjects with malignant tumors it was noted that the development of atherosclerosis in the aorta and coronary arteries is directly dependent on age. As in other groups, lesions in subjects below 40 years of age were primarily fatty streaks; in subjects over 40 years, raised lesions were the predominant finding. Certain differences in the degree of atherosclerosis in the vessels of males and females were noted. Raised lesions in both parts of the aorta were significantly more frequent in males in the fifth, sixth, and seventh decades of life. Only in the young (30–39 years) and very old (70–79 years) age groups were there no differences between males and females. In the coronary arteries these changes were always more extensive in males with malignant tumors than in females. Lipidosis, the mildest type of atherosclerotic change, occupied a greater area of the coronary arteries and abdominal aorta in females than in males. Stenosis of the coronary arteries by more than 50% of the lumen was observed more frequently in males with malignant tumors than in females (Table 17).

The greater severity of atherosclerosis in males than in females suffering from malignant tumors may be explained by the high prevalence and extent of atherosclerotic changes in the entire group and in males in general. This was demonstrated in detail by us in the analysis of atherosclerosis in EHI in chapter 1. In male patients with cancer, the original incidence of atherosclerosis as such was higher than in females. Certainly it cannot be ruled out that these differences are also in part determined by the variations between males and females with regard to the type of tumor. Some data showing the characteristics of the course of atherosclerosis with various types of tumors are presented here.

Table 17. Frequency of Stenosis of the Coronary Arteries in Patients with Malignant Tumors

Age in years	50–59	60–69	70–79
Male	4.7 ± 1.3	24.5 ± 2.6	31.1 ± 3.8
Female	2.9 ± 1.1	5.1 ± 1.3*	13.4 ± 2.6*

* Differences statistically significant ($p \leqslant 0.05$). Frequencies are expressed as a percentage of the number of cases studied.

A group of subjects with malignant tumors was compared with a group of EHI for the prevalence of the various types of atherosclerotic change and for the extent of the area affected.

In both parts of the aorta after the fourth decade of life atherosclerotic changes were generally present; in both groups the coronary arteries were often without change (Table 18). However, the differences between the groups in the prevalence of such afflicted vessels were not statistically significant.

Table 18. Frequency of Coronary Arteries without Atherosclerosis in EHI (1) and in Subjects with Malignant Tumors (2)

Vessels	Groups	Years			
		30–39	40–49	50–59	60–69
Males					
RCA	1	15.9 ± 2.0	5.0 ± 1.3	1.7 ± 0.8	2.1 ± 1.1
	2	20.4 ± 5.7	7.4 ± 1.3	4.3 ± 1.3	1.5 ± 0.8
LADCA	1	3.2 ± 0.9	2.0 ± 0.9	0.4 ± 0.4	0.7 ± 0.7
	2	6.3 ± 3.4	1.5 ± 1.4	0.5 ± 0.4	0.5 ± 0.4
Females					
RCA	1	29.2 ± 4.4	13.4 ± 3.5	10.7 ± 3.2	1.2 ± 1.2
	2	24.4 ± 7.7	18.3 ± 3.7	6.9 ± 1.3	3.5 ± 1.2
LADCA	1	8.5 ± 2.7	5.0 ± 2.2	1.1 ± 1.1	1.2 ± 1.2
	2	18.6 ± 5.9	1.9 ± 1.3	3.4 ± 1.4	1.7 ± 0.8

RCA, right coronary artery; LADCA, LAD coronary artery.

Vessels with only fatty streaks were often seen in both groups in the fourth and fifth decades of life; with age their number diminished, and in the eighth decade of life such vessels were seen only in a small number of cases (aorta, 1.5%; coronary arteries, 4.5–6.5% of cases). In the patients with malignant tumors, vessels with fatty streaks only were noted more frequently than in

EHI. However, the differences were statistically significant only between corresponding groups of males. The cases with fatty streaks and fibrous plaques in the vessels, and similarly with complicated lesions and calcification, were nearly always found somewhat more frequently in EHI than in subjects suffering from malignant tumors, but the differences between the groups were not statistically significant (Table 19).

Table 19. Age-standardized (30–79 years) Indices of Frequency of Vessels with Atherosclerotic Changes in EHI (1) and in Subjects with Malignant Tumors (2)

Vessels	Groups	Lipidosis only	Lipidosis and fibrous plaques	Complicated lesions and calcification
Males				
ThA	1	27.2	46.6	24.8
	2	20.2	51.2	28.2
AA	1	14.0	40.1	45.9
	2	10.3	41.8	47.2
LADCA	1	10.2	60.0	28.7
	2	4.3	62.5	30.4
Females				
ThA	1	29.0	43.5	25.8
	2	27.5	42.7	28.8
AA	1	19.0	44.0	37.2
	2	15.2	44.1	40.6
LADCA	1	16.7	53.8	24.1
	2	14.1	55.2	23.5

ThA, thoracic aorta; AA, abdominal aorta; LADCA, LAD coronary artery.

The comparative characteristics of the average areas occupied by atherosclerotic changes in the aorta and coronary arteries in subjects suffering from malignant tumors and in EHI revealed some differences between the groups. Fatty streaks in the vessels of patients with malignant tumors usually occupied a smaller area than in a group of EHI. Fifty comparisons of atherosclerosis between the groups were conducted according to this index (five vessels in each of the five decades of life, separately for males and females): in 31 comparisons the area with lipidosis in the vessels was greater in healthy people, and in 17 comparisons the area was greater in patients with malignant tumors ($p_{kz} = 0.05$); in two cases there were no differences between the groups. The age-standardized (30–79 years) indices of the area with fatty streaks also decrease in patients with malignant tumors. Moreover, a considerable decrease in the area with lipidosis was noted in the abdominal aorta (both in males and females) and in the LAD coronary artery (only in females).

There were no significant differences between the groups in the extent of raised lesions (fibrous plaques, complicated lesions, and calcification) in the aorta and coronary arteries. No differences were noted with a comparison of the groups by each decade of life and by age-standardized indices (Fig. 15). However, there was a decrease in the area with calcification (particularly in the coronary arteries) in patients with malignant tumors. This was seen in 34 of 44 comparisons in which there were differences between the groups ($p_{kz} < 0.01$). Similarly, it should be noted that in patients with malignant tumors the total area of the coronary arteries with atherosclerotic changes was somewhat smaller than in healthy subjects; in the aorta a reverse tendency was noticed, i.e., in patients with tumors there was some increase in the area with lesions (particularly fibrous plaques).

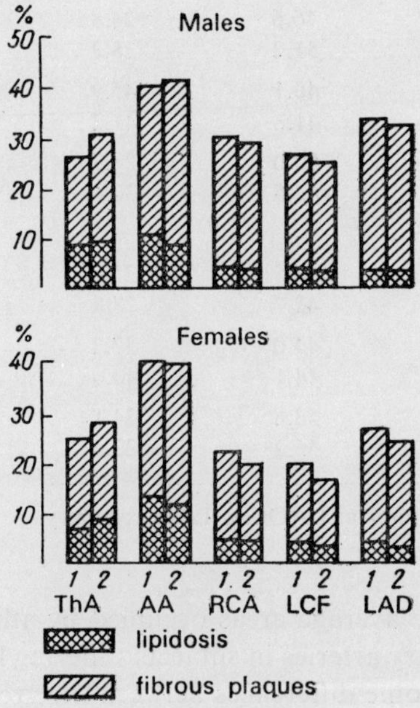

Figure 15. Age-standardized (30–79 years) indices of area with lipidosis and raised lesions in vessels of EHI (*1*) and in patients with malignant tumors (*2*). The ordinate shows the abnormal area as a percentage of the intimal surface of the vessel.

In those dying from the complications of atherosclerosis the total area with atherosclerotic changes and the area with raised lesions (fibrous plaques, complicated lesions, and calcification) were considerably more extensive than in subjects with carcinomas; on the contrary, the area with fatty streaks was greater in the patients with carcinoma. This is most likely due to the more rapid development of raised lesions in persons dying from the complications of atherosclerosis, which by itself decreases the area of intima with fatty streaks. The area with raised lesions and the area with fatty streaks are inversely proportional: with any increase in the area with raised lesions a decrease is observed in the area with fatty streaks.

As is well known, malignant tumors often lead to emaciation. Our studies on the thickness of the subcutaneous fatty tissue in a standard location support this fact. In those with tumors the thickness of the subcutaneous fatty tissue was always less than in healthy people (Table 20).

Table 20. Mean Thickness of Subcutaneous Fatty Tissue (mm) in EHI (1) and in Subjects with Malignant Tumors (2)

Sex	Groups	Years 30–39	40–49	50–59	60–69	70–79
Males	1	13.0	14.6	13.9	15.5	14.1
	2	12.3	12.8	10.6*	10.7*	10.6*
Females	1	23.6	27.0	24.1	12.4	24.5
	2	14.7*	17.0*	20.5*	19.1*	16.5*

* Differences statistically significant ($p \leqslant 0.05$).

With the idea of elucidating the effects of emaciation occurring with malignant tumors on the development of atherosclerosis, we conducted a comparison of the degree of atherosclerosis in subjects with malignant tumors with marked emaciation and without emaciation. The first group included cases in which the thickness of the subcutaneous fatty tissue at the midpoint between the umbilicus and the xiphoid sternum was not more than 5 mm (282 cases); the second group included cases where the thickness of the subcutaneous tissue at this location was 20 mm or more in males and 25 mm or more in females (253 cases).

The differences between the comparable groups in the degree of atherosclerosis in both parts of the aorta were not significant; in females the area in the abdominal aorta with lipidosis was significantly larger in subjects without emaciation. Raised lesions in the aorta occupied practically the same area in both groups (Fig. 16).

The degree of atherosclerosis in the coronary arteries in groups compared by individual decades of life usually did not reveal significant differences in relation to the area with separate types of atherosclerotic change. However, the age-standardized (40–79 years) indices of the area with raised lesions indicate more severe atherosclerotic changes in the group of subjects without emaciation; in females these changes were statistically significant (Fig. 16).

The area with fibrous plaques was greater in non-emaciated subjects (in 21 of 30 comparisons, values were less than 0.05 but greater than 0.01); the age-standardized (40–79 years) indices of the area with fibrous plaques and the area with raised lesions (mainly consisting of fibrous plaques) were also greater in the group of non-emaciated subjects.

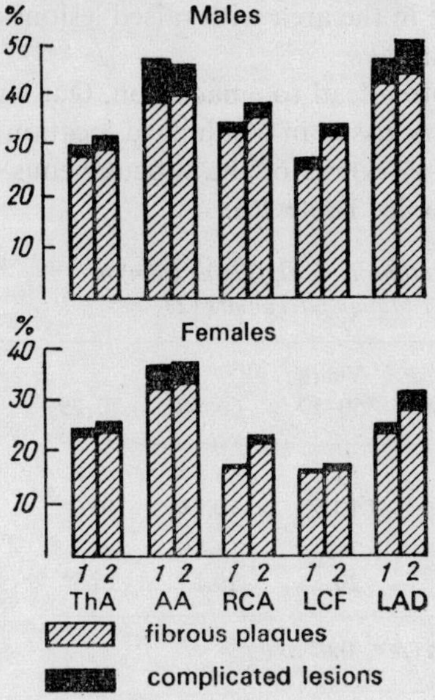

Figure 16. Age-standardized (40–79 years) indices of area with raised lesions in patients with malignant tumors with (*1*) and without emaciation (*2*). Legends as in Fig. 15. ThA, thoracic aorta; AA, abdominal aorta; RCA, right coronary artery; LCF, left circumflex coronary artery; LAD, left anterior descending coronary artery.

Stenosis of the coronary arteries in non-emaciated subjects with malignant tumors was practically always more frequent than in emaciated subjects. The age-standardized (40–79 years) index of the prevalence of stenosis of the coronary arteries in emaciated patients was $16.4 \pm 3.4\%$ and in non-emaciated $27.9 \pm 4.9\%$; in females $3.5 \pm 1.8\%$ and $8.8 \pm 2.8\%$, respectively ($p < 0.05$).

It can be concluded that emaciated patients with malignant tumors have a reduction in the development of atherosclerosis in the coronary arteries. It is interesting that emaciated patients did not differ in the degree of lipidosis in the coronary arteries but did in the area occupied by fibrous plaques. Since fibrous plaques constitute the primary type of raised lesions, the area occupied by raised lesions was also higher in non-emaciated patients.

Let us now examine the differences between the groups in the prevalence of 50% or greater stenosis of the coronary arteries. The low frequency of stenosis in the coronary arteries of emaciated patients with malignant tumors is probably due not only to the reduction in fibrous plaques in these patients but also to smoothing of the plaques. This may be related to resorption of lipid plaques, which we and other investigators noted in emaciated diseases (Wilens, 1947; Kremnev, 1951; Sinapins, 1964; Eilerson and Faber, 1960; Zhdanov *et al.*, 1973). Our histological studies demonstrated that the thickness of the fibrous plaques depends mainly on the quantity of lipid within the plaque and to a small degree on the thickness of the fibrous covering. During a study of the thickness of fibrous plaques in the aortas in 150 males between 50 and 59 years of age who died from malignant tumors, and in EHI, it was established that in emaciated subjects dying from malignant tumors the mean thickness of the aorta and a plaque was rarely more than 2 mm, whereas in healthy people it was 2.5 mm.

The following conclusions can be drawn regarding the characteristics of atherosclerosis in patients with malignant tumors. Although the differences were not statistically significant, some pronounced tendencies were noted in the degree of atherosclerosis in subjects dying from malignant tumors and in EHI. In males and to a lesser degree in females dying from malignant tumors, both parts of the aorta showed tendencies to extensive atherosclerotic changes. This was due to the great extent of fibrous plaques, and in males to complicated lesions as well. The area with calcification in both parts of the aorta was more or less equal in both groups or smaller in subjects with malignant tumors.

In the coronary arteries of males and females the total area with atherosclerotic changes was either the same in both groups or was slightly smaller in most decades of life in subjects with malignant tumors. This was due mainly to the more limited extent of fatty streaks and calcification in the presence of malignant tumors.

A large number of studies carried out by other authors indicate that in patients with malignant tumors the development of atherosclerosis is very slight as compared with a group comprising all other patients. This is quite understandable, since the group comprising all other patients included patients dying from the complications of atherosclerosis, hypertension, chronic nephritis, and other diseases. The group comprising all other patients is nondescript since it includes all these patients. Accordingly, comparisons with this group to evaluate the characteristics and rates of development of atherosclerosis in patients with malignant disease cannot be considered valid.

Therefore, some authors (Parrish, 1961; Katsuki *et al.*, 1964; Giertsen, 1966; Sternby, 1968) compared the degree of atherosclerosis in a group suffering from malignant tumors not with all other deaths, but with a group from which cases of atherosclerotic heart disease, hypertension, diabetes, etc. were excluded, or with a group of victims of accidental death. Here the results obtained are analogous to ours, i.e., differences between the comparable groups in the degree of atherosclerotic process were either slight or altogether absent.

To study the effect of emaciation on the development of atherosclerosis we compared the degree of atherosclerotic process in emaciated and non-emaciated patients. It was found that between these groups there were no differences in the degree of change in both parts of the aorta; in the coronary arteries, however, there was a tendency to a more pronounced change in non-emaciated subjects. If they exist, the minor differences between the groups with different degrees of obesity are possibly due to the relatively rapid appearance of emaciation in patients with malignant tumors.

ATHEROSCLEROSIS AND CARCINOMAS OF THE VARIOUS ORGANS

It was shown above that in subjects with malignant tumors there are no significant differences in the degree of atherosclerosis in this group compared with EHI. However, this does not exclude difference in the development of atherosclerosis in carcinomas of the various organs. The data available in the literature on this problem are limited and contradictory. One group of investigators noted the development of a more severe type of atherosclerosis in patients with lung carcinoma than in patients with carcinomas of other organs (Leites, 1932; Creed *et al.*, 1955; Tiraspol'skaya and Kostyukovskii, 1965; Restrepo *et al.*, 1968), while others (Tichy *et al.*, 1953, Winkelstein *et al.*, 1959, Kumonok, 1967) found no significant differences in the degree of atherosclerosis in patients with lung carcinomas versus those with other carcinomas.

According to Leites (1932), atherosclerosis is rarely observed in cases with a malignant tumor in the female genital organs, pancreas, or liver. Sipovskii and Vlasova (1961) noted that in autopsy studies atherosclerosis has been found most frequently in subjects dying from carcinoma of the pancreas gland, the gall bladder, and the liver (44.3 %), the thyroid gland and the lungs (38.3 %), the kidneys and the urinary bladder (36.8 %). On the other hand, it is rare in malignant tumors of the sex organs (23.5 %). Zschoch (1967) noticed a lower degree of atherosclerosis in all groups of patients with neoplastic growths than in patients with other diseases, but found no such correlation for gastric and gall bladder carcinomas. Kochetov *et al.* (1970) found that in the case of carcinoma of the digestive organs atherosclerosis was rarer than in a control group. The latter was composed of subjects dying from various accidental causes.

We conducted a quantitative evaluation of atherosclerotic lesions in the vessels of patients with common carcinomas: in males with gastric and lung carcinoma; in females with gastric, lung, uterine, ovarian, and breast carcinoma (Table 21). The differences between the groups were not always in the same direction and not always statistically significant in various decades of life, so that difficulties arose in evaluation of the results. These difficulties compelled us to use for comparison the average area with atherosclerotic lesions in a particular decade of life and the age-standardized indices of the area with atherosclerosis, and some nonparametric statistics: criteria of signs (p_{kz}), paired criteria of Wilcoxon (P_t) (Gubler and Genkin, 1973).

In both males and females suffering from gastric carcinoma the total area with atherosclerotic changes and raised lesions in both parts of the aorta proved to be very similar to that noted in EHI. A definite tendency to a lower degree of lipidosis (in both males and females) and calcification (in males) was found in patients with gastric carcinoma.

In the coronary arteries of both males and females suffering from gastric

Table 21. Age and Sex Distribution of Carcinoma Cases

Type of carcinoma	30–39	40–49	Years 50–59	60–69	70–79	Total
Males						
Gastric	13	25	74	82	42	236
Pulmonary	10	19	65	65	26	185
Females						
Gastric	10	25	58	92	36	221
Pulmonary	—	6	14	23	13	56
Uterine	14	35	41	33	21	144
Ovarian	3	18	28	34	6	89
Breast	7	18	34	19	9	87

carcinoma atherosclerotic changes were less extensive than in healthy people. This was true for the total area with atherosclerosis, the total area with raised lesions (Figs. 17 and 18) and for the individual types of lesions.

Out of the 75 comparisons conducted in the corresponding groups of males (three coronary arteries each for five signs and in five decades of life), 51 atherosclerotic changes occupied a greater area in healthy people (in 15 comparisons the differences were statistically significant for particular decades of life). In only 18 patients with gastric carcinoma were the atherosclerotic changes greater than in healthy individuals (the differences were not statistic-

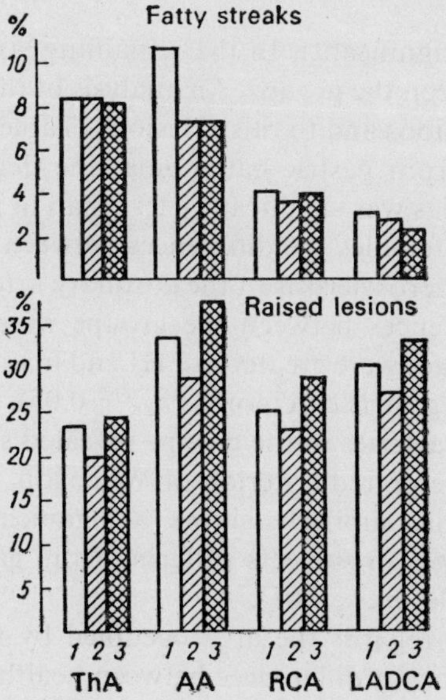

Figure 17. Age-standardized (30–79 years) indices of areas with fatty streaks and raised lesions in vessels of EH males (*1*) and subjects dying from gastric carcinoma (*2*) and lung carcinoma (*3*). Ordinate shows the changed area as percentage of intimal surface of vessel. ThA, thoracic aorta; AA, abdominal aorta; RCA, right coronary artery; LADCA, left anterior descending coronary artery.

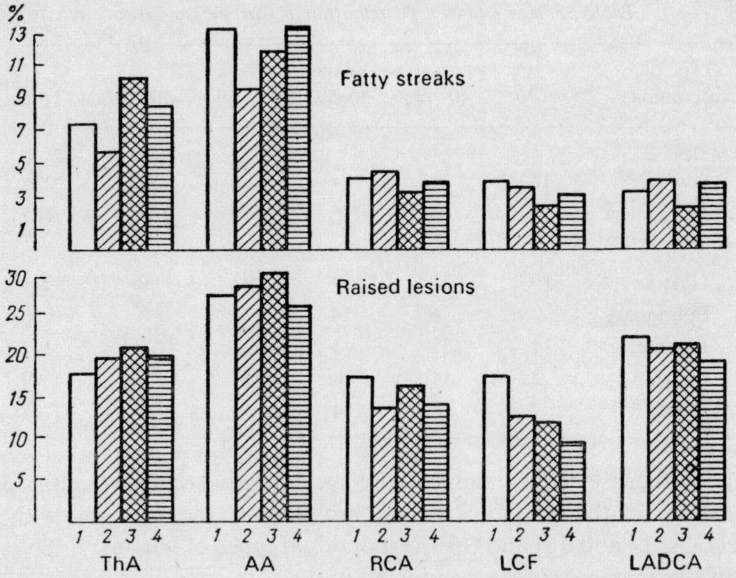

Figure 18. Age-standardized (30–79 years) indices of areas with fatty streaks and raised lesions in vessels of EH females (*1*) and those dying from gastric carcinoma (*2*), carcinoma of the uterus (*3*), and carcinoma of the breast (*4*). Ordinate shows the changed area as percentage of intimal surface of vessel. ThA, thoracic aorta; AA, abdominal aorta; RCA, right coronary artery; LCF, left circumflex coronary artery; LADCA, left anterior descending coronary artery.

ally significant). In the remaining six comparisons there were no differences between the groups. An analysis of the groups with respect to individual types of lesions and to raised lesions (Table 22) demonstrates that in subjects suffering from gastric carcinoma, the degree of atherosclerosis of the coronary arteries was significantly less than in healthy subjects ($p_{kz} = 0.01$).

In females the differences between the corresponding groups in the degree of atherosclerosis in the coronary arteries were significant: of 75 comparisons differences between the groups were present in 67. In 42 comparisons the changes were greater in EHI and in only 25 were they greater in those suffering from gastric carcinoma ($p_{kz} = 0.05$). An analysis of raised lesions in the coronary arteries in the groups revealed similar differences ($p_{kz} = 0.01$) (Fig. 18).

The paired criterion of Wilcoxon, calculated for the total area with raised lesions, similarly shows a significantly smaller area with atherosclerotic changes in subjects suffering from gastric carcinoma (in males $p_t = 0.05$, in females $p_t < 0.01$).

As regards the area occupied by various types of atherosclerotic lesions, significant differences between healthy individuals and those dying from gastric carcinoma were present in calcification of the aorta and coronary arteries (in both males and females) and in lipidosis (only in the coronary arteries of males). These types of lesions occupied a smaller area in patients with gastric carcinoma ($p = 0.05$).

Table 22. Comparisons between EHI and Subjects with Carcinomas

Vessels	Value	Gastric carcinoma		Lung carcinoma		Uterine carcinoma	Breast carcinoma
		Male	Female	Male	Female	Female	Female
Aorta	1*	12	13	5	13	10	14
	2	14	10	21	10	17	9
	p_{kz}	> 0.05	> 0.05	< 0.01	> 0.05	> 0.05	> 0.05
Coronary arteries	1	28	24	14	24	30	34
	2	11	6	20	6	8	4
	p_{kz}	0.01	< 0.01	> 0.05	< 0.01	< 0.01	< 0.01

* (1) number of comparisons showing predominance of lesions in group of EHI; (2) number of comparisons showing predominance of lesions in subjects with various carcinomas; (p_{kz}) criteria of signs that determine the level of statistical significance of differences between groups.

Thus a comparison of atherosclerosis in patients with gastric carcinoma and in EHI indicates a rather low degree of coronary atherosclerosis in the group of patients with gastric carcinoma. This is in agreement with the data of several workers (Sipovskii and Vlasova, 1961; Kochetov *et al.*, 1970), who have also noted the lower frequency and degree of atherosclerosis in patients with gastric carcinoma than in patients with other types of carcinoma and in a control group of EHI.

The low degree of atherosclerosis in the coronary arteries of those suffering from gastric carcinoma is due to significant nutritional disorders leading to emaciation. According to our data the obesity of patients with gastric carcinoma, determined by the thickness of the subcutaneous fatty tissue, was significantly lower than in healthy people (Table 23). The changes in the lipid metabolism of patients with gastric carcinoma, in particular, are characterized by hypocholesteremia and a decreased concentration of lipoproteins in the blood (Medvedeva, 1969). These data correspond with our findings showing a decrease in the area with lipidosis in all the vessels studied in patients with gastric carcinoma. It must be noted that in diseases characterized by emaciation there is a decrease in the area showing accumulations of lipids in macroscopically unchanged intima and in the resorptions of lipids from atherosclerotic plaques. We noticed this during a study of the mechanisms of regression of atherosclerotic process in man (Zhdanov *et al.*, 1973), as have others (Volkova, 1946; Wilens, 1947; Kremnev, 1951).

Table 23. Average Thickness of Subcutaneous Fatty Tissue (mm) in Males with Carcinomas

Age in years	Years 40–49	50–59	60–69	70–79
Healthy	13.0 ± 0.7	14.6 ± 1.0	13.9 ± 0.9	15.5 ± 1.0
Lung carcinoma	10.8 ± 1.5	11.8 ± 2.3	9.3 ± 0.9*	14.0 ± 2.2
Gastric carcinoma	8.2 ± 2.9*	7.7 ± 0.8*	7.6 ± 0.8*	7.0 ± 1.1*

* Differences statistically significant when compared with a group of EHI.

In males suffering from lung carcinoma the area with atherosclerotic changes both in the aorta and in the coronary arteries was greater than in EHI (Fig. 17, Table 22). The great extent of the area with atherosclerosis in patients with lung carcinoma was primarily due to fibrous plaques, which predominated in 21 of 25 comparisons.

Moreover, in 12 comparisons the differences were statistically significant; the criteria of signs also indicate a significantly higher total area with atherosclerosis in patients with lung carcinoma ($p_{kz} < 0.01$). The differences between these groups in the age-standardized indices of the area with raised lesions was also statistically significant as determined by the criterion of signs (only in the aorta) and the paired criterion of Wilcoxon.

Unlike other types of atherosclerotic change, fatty streaks in patients with lung carcinoma occupied a smaller area than in healthy people; the criterion of signs revealed significant differences between the groups in the aorta only in lipidosis ($p_{kz} = 0.05$). Stenosis of the coronary arteries by 50% or more of the lumen was seen more frequently in male patients with lung carcinoma than in healthy people [age-standardized (50–79 years) indices, 25.4% and 17.9%, respectively; $p < 0.05$].

In females suffering from lung carcinoma the degree of atherosclerosis in the aorta was basically the same as in a group of EHI. There were no significant differences in the total area with atherosclerotic changes, in the total area with raised lesions (Table 22), or in individual types of lesions. In the coronary arteries the area with atherosclerotic changes was less in patients with lung carcinoma. In 63 comparisons, differences between the groups were present in 53. In 39 comparisons the changes were greater in the group of EHI, and in only 14 cases were the changes greater in those suffering from lung carcinoma ($p_{kz} < 0.01$).

Marked differences between the groups in raised lesions were also present ($p_{kz} < 0.01$; $p_t < 0.05 > 0.01$).

Thus the results for atherosclerosis of the aorta and coronary arteries in patients with lung carcinoma were different for males and females. The conflicting reports in the literature on the degree of atherosclerosis in patients with lung carcinoma are probably in part related to an inadequate attention to the role of sex in the development of atherosclerosis in these patients. Possibly the conditions and factors responsible for the development of carcinoma of the lung differ for males and females. Variations in the histological structure of carcinoma of the lung in subjects of different sexes support this possibility (Balo, 1957).

An acceleration of atherosclerosis in males dying from lung carcinoma may be related to tobacco smoking, since it is well known that smoking not only increases the risk of lung carcinoma but also favors the development of atherosclerosis (Sedov, 1966; Avtandilov, 1970).

Some investigators (Merrigi, 1960; Moiseenko, 1970) attribute the acceleration of atherosclerosis in lung carcinoma to a rise in the blood cholesterol level. However, according to our data the area with fatty streaks in the vessels studied in patients with carcinoma of the lung was the same or less than in EHI.

In the opinion of several authors (Faconi, 1960; Camus, 1963), patients with lung carcinoma have increased calcification of the arteries resulting from hypercalcemia caused by bone metastases. However, we did not find significant differences in calcification of the arteries between patients with carcinoma of the lung and EHI.

In females with uterine carcinoma there was an intensification of the atherosclerotic process in the aorta as compared with a group of EHI. Of the 50 comparisons conducted between the groups (five signs each in the two parts of the aorta in five decades of life) differences were present in 46 comparisons. In 31 comparisons the lesions were more extensive in patients with uterine carcinoma, and in only 15 in EHI ($p_{kz} < 0.05 > 0.01$). Significant differences in raised lesions between the groups were revealed only with the use of the paired criterion of Wilcoxon ($p_t < 0.05 > 0.01$), which is more sensitive than the criteria of signs.

The degree of atherosclerosis in the coronary arteries was less in patients with uterine carcinoma than in healthy women. This was noted when comparing the groups with all values (the average area of lesions in a particular decade of life, the age-standardized indices of the area with lesions, the criteria of signs, and the paired criteria of Wilcoxon). Considerable differences between the groups were found in the total area with atherosclerotic changes, the total area with raised lesions, and the area with lipidosis, fibrous plaques, and calcification (Fig. 18, Table 22).

In females with breast carcinoma the degree of atherosclerosis in the aorta was the same as in a group of EHI. Among the groups there were no significant differences either in the total area with atherosclerosis or in the area with individual types of lesions. In the coronary arteries of those with breast carcinoma, atherosclerosis was usually of a low degree (Fig. 18, Table 22). In 75 comparisons between the groups (five signs each in three arteries for five decades of life) differences were seen in 66 comparisons. In 53 the changes were more extensive in healthy people, and in 13 changes were extensive in patients with breast carcinoma ($p_{kz} < 0.01$); significant differences between the groups were noted in all measures of atherosclerosis except lipidosis ($p_{kz} =$ 0.05–0.01; p_t for raised lesions < 0.01). The area with calcification in all 15 comparisons was less in patients with carcinoma of the breast ($p_{kz} < 0.01$).

Thus the data indicate a significantly lower degree of atherosclerosis in the coronary arteries of patients with carcinoma of the breast than in healthy people. In the aorta no differences were noted between the groups in the degree of atherosclerosis.

In females with ovarian carcinoma the degree of atherosclerosis in the aorta was usually greater than in healthy subjects. In 40 comparisons (five signs each in the two parts of the aorta for four decades of life) differences between the groups were noted in 38. In 27 comparisons the area with atherosclerotic changes was greater in patients with ovarian carcinoma and in only 13 of the healthy women ($p_{kz} = 0.01$). Most often the difference between the groups was in the area with fibrous plaques and complicated lesions.

The degree of atherosclerosis in the coronary arteries depended on the age of the subjects dying from ovarian carcinoma. In subjects 30 to 49 years old there was a definite tendency to increased atherosclerosis in patients of ovarian carcinoma. In women 50 to 69 years old the degree of atherosclerosis was the same or somewhat less than in all patients with carcinoma (Fig. 19). Calcification of the coronary arteries always occupied a smaller area in subjects dying from ovarian carcinoma.

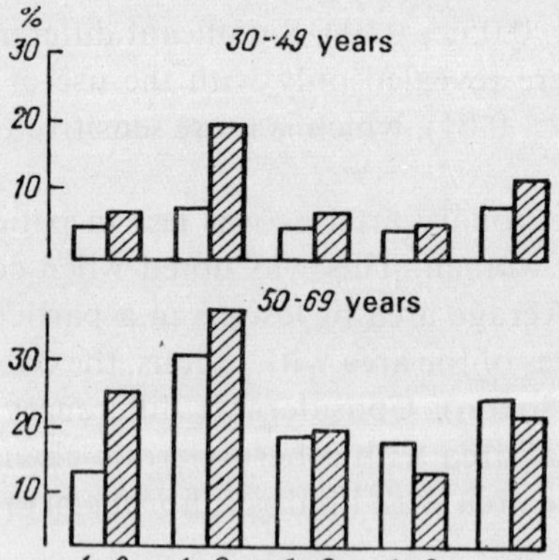

Figure 19. Area with raised lesions in vessels of EH women (*1*) and in subjects dying from ovarian carcinoma (*2*). Ordinate shows the changed area as a percentage of intimal surface of vessel. ThA, thoracic aorta; AA, abdominal aorta; RCA, right coronary artery; LCF, left circumflex coronary artery; LAD, left anterior descending coronary artery.

Development of malignant tumors of the sex organs and breast in females is usually accompanied by various hormonal disorders. The role of sex hormones in the development of atherosclerosis has been demonstrated extensively in a large number of studies. It has been established that estrogens possess a hypocholesteremic and anti-atherosclerotic activity; on the other hand, deficiency of estrogens usually favors the development of atherosclerosis (Rivin and Dimitroff, 1954; Winkelstein *et al.*, 1959; Moses, 1963; Myasnikov, 1969). The peculiarities in the development of atherosclerosis that we observed in subjects dying from carcinoma of the sex organs or breast are to a certain extent related to a change in the hormonal status of these patients. However, it is not possible to exclude completely the effects of other factors on the course of atherosclerosis in such patients.

In many patients with breast carcinoma a rise in the estrogen excretion occurs, which probably also explains the low degree of atherosclerosis in their coronary arteries. This is supported by data from several experimental studies that show that the estrogens affect the development of coronary atherosclerosis to a greater extent than the development of atherosclerosis in the aorta (Myasnikov, 1969). In the literature there are data on the level of estrogens in patients with uterine carcinoma, but they are not as specific. According to one study (Mezinova and Khan, 1972) the level of estrogens in these patients is higher than in a control group, particularly in the climacteric period and in early menopause. The similar course of atherosclerosis in patients with breast and uterine carcinoma is possibly explained by this estrogen elevation.

In patients with ovarian carcinoma the excretion of estrogens may be low or high, depending on the type of tumor; a hypoestrogenic state in such patients may often develop from surgical or radiological treatment of the tumors. In our case, the degree of atherosclerosis in those dying from carcinoma of the ovaries shows an intensification of the atherosclerotic process primarily in ages up to 50 years as compared with a corresponding group of healthy subjects. In subjects above 50 years of age the differences between the comparable groups were present only for atherosclerosis of the aorta. The fact that the differences between the groups in the degree of atherosclerosis were noted more in relatively younger women (up to 50 years of age) suggests that hormonal disorders are among the factors that determine the characteristics of atherosclerosis in patients with ovarian carcinoma.

Thus the degree of atherosclerosis in patients with malignant tumors depends to a certain extent on the type of the tumor. Metabolic, endocrine, and other disorders that occur with carcinoma of various organs determine the development of atherosclerosis in these patients.

5

Atherosclerosis and Cirrhosis of the Liver

Various metabolic disorders, including disorders of cholesterol and lipid metabolism, are frequently observed in liver diseases (Myasnikov, A. L., 1956, 1960, 1965; Grollman, 1962; Myasnikov, L. A., 1962, 1969; Leites, 1966). The role of the liver in the metabolism of cholesterol varies according to the type of animal. In rats and in man, considerably more cholesterol is synthesized in the liver than in rabbits and birds (Grollman, 1962). The cholesterol synthesized in the liver enters the intestinal tract with the bile; a major part of it is then reabsorbed from the intestine into the blood. To understand the pathogenesis of atherosclerosis it must be remembered that the blood cholesterol level is primarily determined by endogenous cholesterol and not by the amount of cholesterol in the diet (Leites, 1966).

Several hormones (for example, hormones of the thyroid gland) affect lipid metabolism mainly through the liver (Myasnikov, L. A., 1969; Fletcher and Myant, 1962; Myasnikov and Pyatenko, 1962).

In liver diseases, in addition to disorders of lipid metabolism, there are often alterations in substances participating in the coagulation and anticoagulation processes. These changes affect the development of atherosclerosis in patients with liver disease (Astrup *et al.*, 1960; Lomazova, 1963; Fletcher *et al.*, 1964; Loginov and Yutanova, 1967).

In various liver diseases and even in different stages of the same disease the disorders in different types of metabolism vary considerably. In most patients with cirrhosis of the liver we find disorders of lipid metabolism found in patients with clinical manifestations of atherosclerosis (Myasnikov, 1956, 1960, 1965; Metelitsa, 1964; Leupold and Kenk, 1965; Warthon, 1965; Il'inskii and Vereshchagina, 1967; Loginov and Yutanova, 1967). In patients with cirrhosis of the liver the total amount of lipids, total phospholipids, and total cholesterol levels in the blood have a tendency to decrease or to be lower than the normal values; in all forms of cirrhosis of the liver the level of cholesterol ester in the blood decreases. The fall in the serum levels of cholesterol and other lipids in cirrhosis of the liver is probably related to a decrease in the synthesis of cholesterol in a diseased liver; in addition, it may be due to hormonal factors such as the rise in the blood level of estrogens since they are not fully inactivated in a cirrhotic liver (Golden and Servinghaus, 1938; Fischer, 1965; Papova, 1965; Il'inskii and Vereshchagina, 1967).

The coagulation and anticoagulation processes in cirrhosis of the liver also affect atherosclerosis. In cirrhosis of the liver consistent changes are noted in these processes that are the opposite of those observed in patients with atherosclerosis. In cirrhosis of the liver the blood heparin level rises, the fibrinogen level falls, and there is high fibrinolytic activity. The degradation of activating enzyme is delayed and the activity of the fibrinolysis inhibitor is reduced (Zaitsev and Ananchenko, 1967).

The data on the fibrinogen level in the blood in patients with cirrhosis of the liver are contradictory. Brodsky and Dennis (1966) observed a fall in the blood fibrinogen level, while Loginov and Yutanova (1967) observed a rise. The increase in the level of fibrinogen in the blood was explaincd by Yutanova as a nonspecific reaction resulting from cirrhotic activity and the inflammatory process in the intrahepatic ducts. She also noted an inverse relationship between the level of fibrinogen in the blood and the degree of fibrinolytic activity; the lowest fibrinolytic activity was found in primary biliary cirrhosis when a very high level of fibrinogen was present and the highest fibrinolytic activity accompanied a very low level of fibrinogen in patients with postnecrotic cirrhosis.

There are few pathological studies of atherosclerosis in patients with cirrhosis of the liver. The studies are almost exclusively based on the analysis of autopsy forms. In all the studies known to us it has been found that severe forms of atherosclerosis are rarely seen in patients with cirrhosis of the liver (Rosenthal, 1934; Gandzha, 1961; Creed *et al.*, 1955; Restrepo *et al.*, 1968; Gandzha *et al.*, 1971). Zschoch (1964, 1967), on the basis of an analysis of voluminous pathological material, concluded that atherosclerosis is rarely found in patients with cirrhosis of the liver, and when present it is of a mild degree. According to Zschoch, cirrhosis of the liver is very frequently associated with diseases like diabetes, endocarditis, and gallstones, and rarely with hypertension, myocardial infarction, and severe cardiosclerosis.

It has been demonstrated in isolated studies (Lukash and Kaganovich, 1965; Abdullaev *et al.*, 1974) that certain characteristics of the atherosclerotic process depend on the type of pathology in the liver and bile ducts. In patients with gallstones (without inflammation) atherosclerosis is frequent and more extensive than in patients without diseases of the liver or bile ducts. In the opinion of these authors this relationship occurs because both diseases (atherosclerosis and gallstone disease) are related to disorders of lipid metabolism. In other liver diseases, including cirrhosis of the liver, the authors failed to demonstrate a significant difference in the frequency and degree of atherosclerosis compared with that in a control group (autopsy forms for victims of fatal accidents). Hirst *et al.* (1965) obtained interesting data when they studied chronic alcoholism with or without cirrhosis of the liver. It was found that in chronic alcoholism without cirrhosis of the liver the frequency of severe narrowing and thrombosis of the coronary arteries and myocardial infarction was the same as in control groups. However, in the case of chronic alcoholism with cirrhosis of the liver the above phenomena were rarely noted; i.e., it appears that cirrhosis of the liver protects against coronary heart disease.

Comparison of the frequency and degree of atherosclerosis in subjects dying from cirrhosis of the liver with the material from all other autopsies in Leningrad demonstrated that severe atherosclerosis was rarely noted in patients with cirrhosis of the liver (Il'inskii and Vereshchagina, 1967). Nevertheless, in some patients with cirrhosis of the liver there is a sharply pronounced, extensive atherosclerosis; it is possible that in some of these cases cirrhosis of the liver developed in the presence of marked atherosclerosis.

During the analysis of autopsy forms, Loginov and Yutanov (1967) found signs of advanced atherosclerosis in the aorta and coronary arteries in only 3 of 32 patients with cirrhosis of the liver. In 20 cases they found moderately pronounced atherosclerotic changes in the aorta without any lesions in the coronary arteries.

Some authors (MacDonald and Mallory, 1958) indicate the great rarity of coronary atherosclerosis in cirrhosis of the liver, although atherosclerosis of the aorta in this disease may be very pronounced. Hall *et al.* (1953), in a study of the autopsy forms of 782 cases of portal cirrhosis, noted that in subjects with cirrhosis of the liver up to 55 years of age coronary atherosclerosis of moderate or severe degree was twice as rare as among other patients. The comparative rarity of severe coronary atherosclerosis in cirrhosis of the liver also explains the very rare development of myocardial infarction in these patients. According to Howell and Manion (1960), only 32 cases of myocardial infarction were observed in 639 cases of cirrhosis of the liver (4.9%). In the remaining group of patients myocardial infarction was observed in 20.2%; even in patients with diabetes mellitus combined with cirrhosis of the liver myocardial infarction was as rare as in patients with cirrhosis of the liver without diabetes.

In those with cirrhosis of the liver there are frequently nonatherosclerotic lesions of the myocardium (known as myocardiosis), which on the basis of ECG are often diagnosed as the manifestations of an atherosclerotic disease (Lunseth *et al.*, 1958; Nielson and Kessing, 1965). Therefore reliable data on the prevalence and on the degree of the atherosclerotic process in cirrhosis of the liver can be obtained only from clinicopathological findings.

Data showing the rarity of myocardial infarction in cirrhosis of the liver were obtained on the basis of comparison of the prevalence of myocardial infarction in patients with cirrhosis of the liver and subjects with other diseases; among the latter, patients with atherosclerosis and hypertension constitute a major part. According to Grosse (1964), who collected 1,892 cases of cirrhosis of the liver from the literature, myocardial infarction in cirrhosis of the liver was found in 3.5% of cases without autopsy, but in 10% with autopsy. If the prevalence and fatalities from myocardial infarction in large groups of people without cirrhosis of the liver (healthy and diseased) are compared with patients with cirrhosis of the liver, no significant differences are found. Grosse concludes that there is not a difference between the prevalence of myocardial infarction in those with cirrhosis of the liver and other subjects. He also states that it is not valid to compare the prevalence of various phenomena on the basis of hospital autopsy records alone because of the special selection involved.

The pathological finding that severe degrees of atherosclerosis are rarely seen in patients with cirrhosis of the liver has also been confirmed experimentally. In rabbits experimental cirrhosis produced by carbon tetrachloride retarded the development of atherosclerosis (Metelitsa, 1964; Fischer, 1965). In these experiments changes also occurred in lipid metabolism: hypocholesteremia, a fall in the cholesterol phospholipid ratio, and a fall in the level of β lipoproteins were observed.

Fischer (1965) attributes the retarding effect of cirrhosis of the liver on the development of atherosclerosis to an excessive accumulation of estrogens in the organism. The data indicate that in cirrhosis of the liver there are considerable changes in lipid metabolism, alterations in the level of estrogens in the blood, and disorders in coagulation, which probably also intensify the retarding effect of cirrhosis of the liver on the development of atherosclerosis.

It should be remembered that patients with cirrhosis of the liver have a tendency to develop hypotension (Loyke, 1955; Myasnikov, 1956; Loginov and Yutanova, 1967). This is also considered to be one of the factors favoring the slower development of the atherosclerotic process. To study the characteristics of the development of atherosclerosis we investigated the aortas and coronary arteries of 203 patients dying with cirrhosis (Table 24). The cirrhosis was characterized as postnecrotic, atrophic, or annular on the basis of pathological findings. Cases of cirrhosis of the liver due to chronic alcoholism and biliary cirrhosis were not included in the analysis because of their small number. Cases combined with several diseases (for example, cases with

Table 24. Age and Sex Distribution of Patients with Cirrhosis of the Liver

Age in years	10–19	20–29	30–39	40–49	50–59	60–69	Total
Males	5	7	21	27	37	24	121
Females	2	4	10	19	26	21	82

hypertension, diabetes mellitus, neoplastic growths, etc.), were also excluded since each of the diseases might influence the development of the atherosclerotic process.

The main changes with age of the atherosclerotic process in the aorta and coronary arteries of those suffering from cirrhosis of the liver were the same as those observed in other groups. In all the vessels, with each decade of life there was a rise in the total area with atherosclerotic changes, and also a rise in the area occupied by fibrous plaques, complicated lesions, and calcification. The area occupied by fatty streaks increased in the aorta only up to the fourth or fifth decade of life, and then gradually decreased; in the coronary arteries fatty streaks occupied a small area (2–4.5% of the intimal surface), the average extent varying little with age.

COMPARISON OF ATHEROSCLEROSIS IN PATIENTS WITH CIRRHOSIS OF THE LIVER AND IN EHI

Beginning with the third decade of life, in practically all cases in both groups, atherosclerotic changes were found in the aorta. The major differences between the groups were the frequency of fatty streaks alone and complicated lesions and/or calcification in the aorta.

The comparative data for the groups in individual decades of life, as well as the age-standardized indices (Table 25), showed that cases with only fatty streaks in both parts of the aorta were more frequent in EHI, and complicated lesions and/or calcification were more frequent in patients with cirrhosis of the liver. In both parts of the aorta the differences between the groups in the frequency of fatty streaks in combination with fibrous plaques were insignificant.

Unlike the aorta data, in the coronary arteries of the groups atherosclerotic changes were absent in some cases. Coronary arteries without atherosclerosis were quite frequently noted in males with cirrhosis of the liver; in females these differences between the groups were absent, and an unchanged right coronary artery was observed more frequently in EHI. Early atherosclerotic changes, particularly coronary arteries with fatty streaks only, were found more frequently in EHI. Moreover, in the groups of males the differences in the right coronary artery and the LAD coronary artery were significant (Table 25). Fatty streaks in combination with fibrous plaques were also seen more frequently in EHI. In males the differences were significant in respect to both branches of the left coronary artery.

Atherosclerotic changes characterizing the most severe degree of the atherosclerotic process—complicated lesions and/or calcification—were present more frequently in the coronary arteries of patients with cirrhosis of the liver. In males in all the arteries, and in females in the left circumflex coronary artery, the differences between the groups were statistically significant in relation to age-standardized indices (Table 25).

Table 25. Age-standardized (30–69) Indices of Frequency of Atherosclerotic Changes in EHI (1) and in Patients with Cirrhosis of the Liver (2)

Type of changes	Groups	ThA	AA	RCA	LCCA	LADCA
Males						
No change	1	—	—	6.2	9.8	1.6
	2	—	—	13.2*	17.4*	7.0*
Lipidosis only	1	33.6	17.1	22.7	21.3	11.4
	2	22.4*	14.5	12.5*	17.1	4.2*
Lipidosis and fibrous plaques	1	48.2	46.6	54.8	58.1	65.6
	2	50.9	42.2	48.8	48.5*	55.9*
Complicated lesions and/or calcification	1	17.8	36.2	16.3	10.8	21.5
	2	26.7*	43.3	25.5*	17.0*	32.8*
Females						
No change	1	—	—	13.6	12.8	3.9
	2	—	—	6.8*	14.4	1.8
Lipidosis only	1	36.6	23.8	35.6	38.9	22.5
	2	29.8	9.8*	32.8	31.9	17.8
Lipidosis and fibrous plaques	1	49.0	49.6	41.2	42.5	58.3
	2	48.6	53.6	48.3	40.2	57.8
Complicated lesions and/or calcification	1	14.2	26.6	9.6	5.8	15.2
	2	22.2	36.5	12.1	3.5*	22.6

ThA, thoracic aorta; AA, abdominal aorta; RCA, right coronary artery; LCCA, left circumflex coronary artery; LADCA, left anterior descending coronary artery.

* Differences statistically significant ($p \leqslant 0.05$).

COMPARISON OF ATHEROSCLEROTIC AREAS IN EHI AND CIRRHOSIS PATIENTS

The total area with atherosclerotic changes in both parts of the aorta in males and females of the two groups differed little or was smaller in patients with cirrhosis of the liver (Fig. 20). Some differences between the groups in the total extent of atherosclerotic changes in the aorta were related primarily to the small extent of fatty streaks in the aorta of patients with cirrhosis of the liver. This is confirmed by comparing the groups in the area of raised lesions

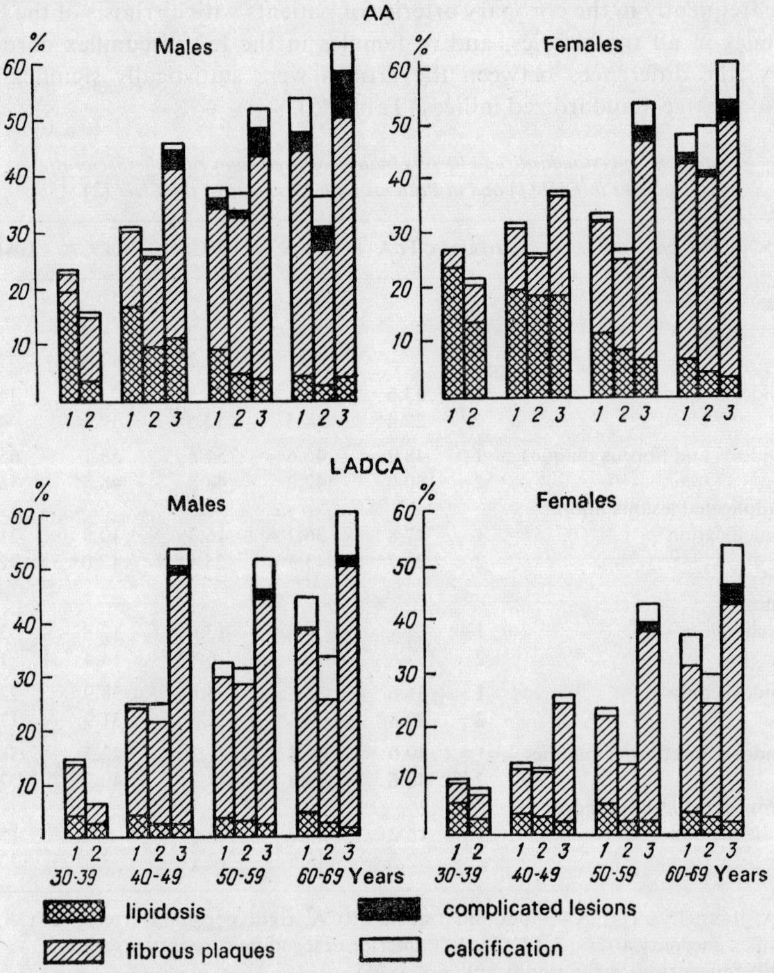

Figure 20. Changes in the area with atherosclerotic changes in the abdominal aorta and LAD coronary artery. *1*, healthy subjects; *2*, patients with cirrhosis of the liver; *3*, subjects dying from complications of atherosclerosis. Ordinate shows abnormal area as a percentage of the intimal surface of vessel.

only, since such comparisons do not reveal significant differences in the degree of atherosclerosis in the aorta in the individual decades of life or in standardized indices (Table 26).

The total area with atherosclerotic changes and also the area with raised lesions in the coronary arteries of males and females with cirrhosis of the liver was usually less than in healthy people (Fig. 20). The differences between the groups increased with age. In the fourth and fifth decades of life, the differences for raised lesions were statistically significant in only one of 12 com-

Table 26. Age-standardized (30–69 years) Indices of Atherosclerotic Areas in EHI (1) and Cirrhosis Patients (2)

Changes	Groups	ThA	AA	RCA	LCCA	LADCA
Males						
Lipidosis	1	9.7	12.1	4.3	3.5	3.0
	2	8.2	7.1*	3.0*	2.3*	2.0*
Raised lesions	1	13.1	24.3	20.7	17.9	25.7
	2	15.2	21.7	15.9*	14.2	21.5*
Females						
Lipidosis	1	8.0	15.6	4.1	3.8	3.7
	2	9.5	11.3*	3.1	2.3*	2.7*
Raised lesions	1	11.0	19.8	12.1	11.2	16.3
	2	11.9	17.5	9.2*	8.9	13.4*

ThA, thoracic aorta; AA, abdominal aorta; RCA, right coronary artery; LCCA, left circumflex coronary artery; LADCA, left anterior descending coronary artery. Abnormal area given as a percentage of the intimal surface of vessel.

* Differences statistically significant ($p \leqslant 0.05$).

parisons. In the sixth and seventh decades of life these differences were present in two-thirds of the comparisons conducted. Age-standardized indices of the area of the coronary arteries with raised lesions were always less in patients with cirrhosis of the liver. These differences were statistically significant for the right coronary artery and for the LAD coronary artery.

AGE-RELATED CHANGES IN ATHEROSCLEROSIS

There were no significant differences between the groups in the areas with fatty streaks in the thoracic aorta; the differences were also not unidirectional. In all other vessels the area with fatty streaks was generally smaller in patients with cirrhosis, and the differences between the groups were often statistically significant both in the individual decades of life and in the age-standardized index (Table 26).

There were no significant differences between the groups in the area with fibrous plaques in the thoracic aorta, although during comparison of the groups in isolated decades of life the area was somewhat higher in patients with liver cirrhosis. In the abdominal aorta and all the coronary arteries fibrous plaques usually occupied a smaller area in patients with cirrhosis of the liver. Comparisons in isolated decades of life yielded statistically significant differences in every third comparison. Age-standardized (30–69 years) indices of the area with fibrous plaques also showed a smaller area with fibrous plaques in patients with cirrhosis of the liver. Maximal differences were noted between the groups of males (Fig. 21).

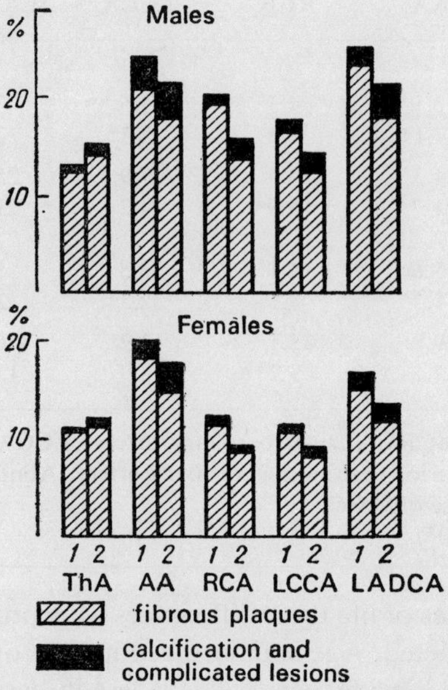

Figure 21. Age-standardized (30–69 years) indices of area with raised lesions in vessels of EHI (*1*) and patients with cirrhosis of the liver (*2*). ThA, thoracic aorta; AA, abdominal aorta; RCA, right coronary artery; LCCA, left circumflex coronary artery; LADCA, left anterior descending coronary artery.

Complicated lesions were equal or slightly more extensive in the group of patients with cirrhosis of the liver than in EHI.

The area with calcification in all the vessels of patients with cirrhosis of the liver was often greater than in EHI (Fig. 20, Table 27). The greater extent of calcification in patients with cirrhosis of the liver was frequently observed in the presence of a smaller area of fibrous plaques than that found in the group of EHI. Therefore, the ratio of the area with fibrous plaques to the area with calcification was considerably less in the patients with cirrhosis of the liver than in healthy people (Table 28). Stenosis of the coronary arteries by 50 % or more was seen only in subjects over age 50 in the group of patients with cirrhosis of the liver. In males the differences between groups in the frequency of this stenosis in the coronary arteries were insignificant (in patients 50 to 69 years of age stenosis was found in 8.2 % of cases; in healthy subjects, in 8.2 %); in females the differences were greater (4.4 % and 9.2 %, respectively).

Macroscopic examination of the vessels of subjects with cirrhosis of the liver frequently revealed calcification of atherosclerotic plaques, while the total area with atherosclerotic changes was small. In some vessels practically all plaques had some degree of calcification (Fig. 22).

The degree of atherosclerosis in the thoracic aorta as indicated by the area with raised lesions in patients with cirrhosis of the liver differs little from the degree of change in healthy people.

Table 27. Age-standardized (40–69 years) Indices of Calcification in Vessels of EHI (1) and Cirrhosis Patients (2)

Vessels	Group	Calcification frequency		Calcification area	
		Male	Female	Male	Female
ThA	1	15.9	12.5	0.5	0.4
	2	21.1	23.6*	0.8	0.7
AA	1	38.7	30.8	2.7	1.8
	2	46.2	39.5	3.2	3.3*
RCA	1	17.3	11.8	1.5	0.9
	2	29.2	16.1	2.9*	1.0
LCCA	1	13.1*	7.9	1.4	0.7
	2	22.7	14.9*	2.4	1.0
LADCA	1	23.2	18.7	2.8	2.2
	2	42.8*	27.0	4.5*	2.6

ThA, thoracic aorta; AA, abdominal aorta; RCA, right coronary artery; LCCA, left circumflex coronary artery; LADCA, left anterior descending coronary artery.

* Differences statistically significant ($p \leqslant 0.05$). Frequency is percentage of observations, and area is percentage of intimal surface of vessel.

Table 28. Area Ratios between Fibrous Plaques and Calcification in EHI and in Cirrhosis Patients

Vessels	Abdominal aorta				Left anterior descending coronary artery			
Age	50–59		60–69		50–59		60–69	
Sex	M	F	M	F	M	F	M	F
Healthy	17.2	18.9	6.5	9.3	11.2	15.2	6.4	5.6
Cirrhosis patients	3.0	10.0	4.5	4.9	9.6	5.2	3.0	4.0

Generally the abdominal aorta, but particularly the coronary arteries, show less pronounced atherosclerosis in patients with cirrhosis of the liver than in healthy people. The differences between the groups in the degree of atherosclerosis in the coronary arteries (total area with changes, area with raised lesions) were often statistically significant.

One of the special features of atherosclerosis in cirrhosis patients is that the extent of fatty streaks is considerably less than in healthy people. This was

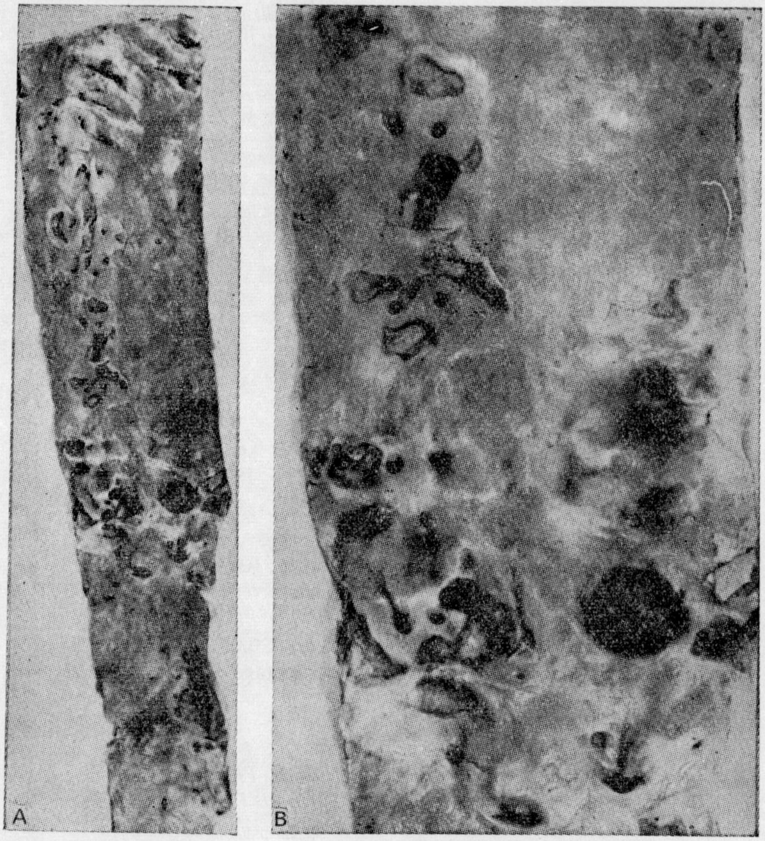

Figure 22. Calcification of most atherosclerotic plaques in the aorta of a 66-year-old female with atrophic cirrhosis of the liver. *A*, the entire descending aorta; *B*, thoracic aorta at higher magnification. Calcified plaques are dark gray in color.

observed in all vessels except the thoracic aorta. The differences between the groups in the total area with atherosclerotic changes are to a considerable degree due to the smaller extent of fatty streaks in the patients with cirrhosis of the liver. In both parts of the aorta no significant differences were found in the area with fibrous plaques. However, in the coronary arteries the area with fibrous plaques was smaller in patients with cirrhosis of the liver.

Our findings show that atherosclerosis in patients with cirrhosis of the liver also has some unique features such as intense calcification of the atherosclerotic plaques. In a group of patients with cirrhosis calcification of the aorta and coronary arteries is more frequent and usually greater in extent than in healthy people. There were no differences between the groups in other types of changes such as complicated lesions.

The characteristics of atherosclerosis in cirrhosis patients to some degree coincide with the data available in the literature. From our data and also from the materials of other workers (Creed *et al.*, 1955; Zschoch, 1964, 1965; Lukash and Kaganovich, 1965; Il'inskii and Vereshchagina, 1967; Loginov and Yutanova, 1967) it appears that severe degrees of atherosclerosis are rarely seen in patients with cirrhosis of the liver. This conclusion has been drawn by most workers on the basis of comparisons of the degree of atherosclerosis (from autopsy records) in a group of such patients with the degree of atherosclerosis in all other patients. In the latter there were cases of hypertension, atherosclerosis, chronic nephritis, diabetes mellitus—diseases where atherosclerotic changes were more pronounced. During such comparisons the degree of atherosclerosis in those suffering from cirrhosis of the liver was always less than in the group comprising all other patients. Only a few studies (Lukash and Kaganovich, 1965; Restrepo *et al.*, 1968) that compared the degree of atherosclerosis in patients with cirrhosis of the liver with that in EHI failed to establish any differences between the groups in the degree of atherosclerosis. In our study the differences between analogous groups in both parts of the aorta were not marked, although there was a tendency toward reduced atherosclerosis in the abdominal aorta in patients with cirrhosis of the liver. In the coronary arteries this tendency was more pronounced. Our data confirm the observations of MacDonald and Mallory (1958) that in cirrhosis of the liver a severe degree of atherosclerosis of the coronary arteries is rarely seen, although atherosclerosis of the aorta may be fairly pronounced.

Some authors have noted the rarity of coronary atherosclerosis and myocardial infarction in patients with cirrhosis of the liver (Hall *et al.*, 1953; Howell and Manion, 1960).

As indicated previously, the inhibitory effect of cirrhosis on the development of atherosclerosis is related to disorders in lipid metabolism, increased levels of estrogens, disorders of the coagulation and anticoagulation processes, and hypotension. These factors probably explain the rather slow development of atherosclerosis in the coronary arteries of patients with cirrhosis of the liver compared to other people. The factors have considerably less effect on the development of atherosclerosis in the aorta.

One of the special features of atherosclerosis that we observed in patients with cirrhosis of the liver is the intense calcification of the atherosclerotic plaques. This is observed even when the total area with atherosclerosis and the area with fibrous plaques are smaller than in healthy individuals. These data indicate that there is not a strict parallelism between the degree of atherosclerosis and calcification in all patients. This is easily demonstrable by determination of the ratio of area with fibrous plaques to area with calcification. This ratio is considerably lower in patients with cirrhosis of the liver than in healthy people.

Intense calcification of the vessels in cirrhosis of the liver may be related to changes in salt and water metabolism that accompany cirrhosis. Similarly, it is possible that dystrophic changes may occur in the vessels. Romanenko (1965) studied the role of the liver in the metabolism of calcium and found that the liver is capable of storing the calcium that enters it from the intestine. This calcium is then excreted in the bile in a concentration higher than in the blood. In cirrhosis of the liver there is a disorder of vitamin metabolism, in particular vitamin D metabolism, which may affect calcium metabolism. Hass *et al.* (1969) showed that in rabbits with experimental cirrhosis of the liver and hypercholesterolemia generalized calcified atherosclerosis is produced with the regular administration of 12,500 units of vitamin D. But in the absence of cirrhosis regular administration of 50,000 units of vitamin D is necessary to produce the same effect.

There may be other factors that contribute to the intense deposition of calcium in fibrous plaques in patients with cirrhosis of the liver. Some investigators have observed osteoporosis in these patients (Colleson *et al.*, 1965), which can lead to an increased concentration of calcium in the blood and favors its accumulation in a vessel wall. The osteoporosis may be due to various types of endocrine disorders, which are often present in cirrhosis. For instance, Stupina (1950) has demonstrated that hyperplasia of the parathyroid glands occurs in patients with cirrhosis of the liver.

6

Atherosclerosis and Rheumatic Heart Disease

The problem of the interrelation of atherosclerosis and rheumatic heart disease (RHD) has long attracted the attention of researchers. The interest in this problem has increased because a considerable number of patients with RHD now live beyond the age of 50 when atherosclerotic lesions of the coronary arteries become frequent. According to the pathological data of Permyakov and Podol'skii (1964) 53.9% of 1,150 patients with valvular heart disease were over 50 years of age. The rise in the number of patients with RHD in middle and old age is associated with the frequent combination of RHD with atherosclerosis (Spektor, 1967; Sumarakov and Fokina, 1967; Shamarin, 1968).

Data concerning the characteristics of atherosclerosis in patients with RHD are contradictory. Most researchers have failed to find intensification of atherosclerosis in such patients (Gross and Oppenheimer, 1936; Wartman and Hellerstein, 1948; Anichkov, 1953; Doerr, 1963; Moses, 1963; Spektor, 1967). Gross and Oppenheimer noted a combination of coronary atherosclerosis and RHD in only 0.91% of cases in an analysis of 3,264 autopsies; the coronary arteries in patients with RHD as a rule showed little change. Voronkov (1967) studied 26 cases with RHD and found some intensification of atherosclerosis in the aorta and coronary arteries compared with healthy people, but the differences were not statistically significant. Chebotarev (1959) noted frequent lesions of the coronary arteries in RHD, particularly of the fine branches, but sclerosis of the main trunks of the coronary arteries was relatively rare. Ochkur *et al.* (1967) noted mild or moderately pronounced atherosclerosis in 65% of subjects dying from RHD. These authors noticed that severe degrees of atherosclerosis most frequently developed in combination with hypertension, rheumatic endocarditis, and specific meso-aortitis. The data of Ochkur *et al.*, which indicate that severe forms of atherosclerosis develop in combination with rheumatic endocarditis, contradict the above-mentioned findings.

Histological and histochemical research (Chiari, 1928; Talałaev, 1929; Klinge, 1933; Kraevskii, 1937; Skvortsov, 1938; Strukov, 1961) has demonstrated that in RHD severe changes are observed in the connective tissue of the heart muscle and vessels. The various changes in the vascular wall observed in patients with RHD, in the opinion of a number of investigators, also favor the development of the atherosclerotic process (Klinge, 1933; Egorov, 1936; Holle, 1943; Mitin, 1966; Strukov and Beglaryan, 1963). Schettler (1955), Nepryakhin (1966), Shultz and Klinge (1933), Holle and Nierade (1963), and Nepryakhin and Akhmetzyanov (1966) have also described the intensifying effect of RHD on the development of atherosclerosis.

Although generalized lesions of the connective tissue of the vascular wall are observed in RHD, the degree of change in different vessels is highly variable. Most often only the smaller vessels are affected (Talalaev, 1929; Klinge, 1933; Karsner and Bayless, 1934; Kraevskii, 1937, 1943; Skvortsov, 1938; Horn, 1959; Strukov, 1961; Mitin, 1966; Strukov and Beglaryan, 1963). More extensive changes are observed in the coronary arteries, followed by the aorta, the renal arteries, the major arteries of the brain and the extremities. In the walls of large vessels the specific changes are localized mainly in the region of the vasa vasorum; the changes are usually nonspecific in the intima and inner portion of media of the major arteries.

In a macroscopic study of atherosclerosis some workers (Wang and Hu, 1957; Moses, 1963) observed different effects of rheumatic disease on the development of the atherosclerotic process in the aorta and coronary arteries. In the aorta atherosclerosis was more pronounced in patients with rheumatic disease than in a control group; the situation was reversed when the coronary arteries were considered. In cases with rheumatic disease the changes in the aorta are observed mostly in the adventitia, but there are also changes in other layers of the aortic wall (Shultz and Klinge, 1933; Morehead, 1965; Mitin, 1966; Nepryakhin, 1966). The changes are often so marked that they are known as rheumatic aortitis. Occasionally they are accompanied by the development of an aortic aneurysm (Holle, 1943; Kushnir and Kozachuk, 1966; Spasskaya, 1967; Kettler, 1970).

Rheumatic changes in the aorta are generally localized to the ascending part of the thoracic aorta and the arch of the aorta; they are rarely found in the abdominal aorta (Libiyainen, 1963).

From the data available in the literature, Mitin (1966) described the pathological changes in the arterial walls in rheumatic disease such as swelling and mucus formation, i.e., so-called fibrinoid swelling and necrosis. There is gradual cellular proliferation in the intima and infiltration of lymphocytes and histiocytes into the walls and perivascular connective tissue. In some cases typical Aschoff-Talalaev nodules are noted; often the vascular lesions are nonspecific in nature.

The so-called latent period of rheumatic diseases is frequently characterized by nonspecific changes in the vessels, which are known in Mitin's terminology as sclerosis characteristic of age or arteriosclerotic changes (the latter are often more extensive than in a control group).

Other factors also affect the development of atherosclerosis in rheumatic disease. Changes in lipid and protein metabolism, the coagulation and anticoagulation systems, the endocrine system, and hypoxia may all cause changes in atherosclerosis.

The changes in lipid metabolism differ depending on the stage (active or latent) of the rheumatic disease. Acute rheumatic disease is accompanied by a fall in the blood cholesterol level, a fall in the level of α-lipoproteins, a rise in the level of β-lipoproteins, and less esterification of cholesterol (Mikunis, 1963; Petrovskii *et al.*, 1972).

The changes in coagulation factors in rheumatic disease are a fall in the fibrinolytic activity of the blood, a rise in the fibrinogen level, and a decrease in the level of free heparin (Syurin, 1966; Grigor'eva, 1967). The above changes predispose these patients to the development of thrombus. Possibly they are also important for the development of atherosclerotic changes, particularly in the presence of simultaneous changes in the arterial wall.

In rheumatic heart disease there are often disorders of the endocrine glands. In RHD patients there are signs of failure of the adrenal cortex as indicated by both morphological (Strukov, 1961; Mironov, 1963) and biochemical (Evnina *et al.*, 1967) studies.

Some authors noticed the frequent combination of rheumatic heart disease with thyroid disease (thyrotoxicosis) (Abaeva, 1967). It has been suggested that rheumatic heart disease predisposes to the development of thyrotoxicosis (see chapter 9).

Thus the available data are contradictory regarding changes in the degree of atherosclerosis in rheumatic heart disease. A number of researchers have observed intensification of atherosclerosis in rheumatic heart disease, especially in the aorta. They related this to the rheumatic changes in the vessels (aortitis, arteritis). These changes, specific and frequently nonspecific, favor the rapid development of atherosclerosis, which has been designated by some authors as "secondary" atherosclerosis (Nepryakhin, 1966) or as rheumatic arteriosclerosis (Mitin, 1966). In our opinion this nomenclature is incorrect, since the atherosclerotic changes in the aorta and other major arteries usually do not differ from those found in other diseases and conditions with nonspecific changes in the vessels. In patients with rheumatic disease other factors, such as changes in lipid and protein metabolism, coagulation and anticoagulation systems, endocrine function and hypoxia, probably also affect the development of atherosclerosis.

In view of the contradictions in the literature on the effect of rheumatic heart disease on the development of atherosclerosis we conducted a morphometric study of atherosclerosis in 458 patients with RHD (Table 29). Most patients died from cardiac failure developed from rheumatic valvular disease. On autopsy active RHD was present in only a small number of cases. Some patients with RHD who actually died in accidents (mostly from trauma) were included in the cases studied.

Table 29. Age and Sex Distribution of RHD Patients

Age in years	20–29	30–39	40–49	50–59	60–69	Total
Male	26	55	53	52	15	201
Female	30	48	53	76	50	257

All the cases of a combination of RHD with other diseases that might influence the development of atherosclerosis were excluded from the analysis; similarly, cases with isolated aortic valvular disease and acute infective endocarditis were not included in the study. The study of the atherosclerotic changes in patients with RHD included patients in the third through the seventh decade of life.

In patients with rheumatic heart disease, as in other groups of patients, a relationship is present between the degree of atherosclerosis and age. The total area with atherosclerotic changes and the area with raised lesions, i.e., fatty streaks, complicated lesions, and calcification, increased with age. The area with fatty streaks increased in the aorta up to the third or fourth decade of life, then gradually diminished, and in the seventh decade occupied only 4 to 6% of the intimal surface. In the coronary arteries the area with lipidosis changed little from one decade to another, rarely occupying more than 4 to 5% of the intimal surface. The total area with atherosclerotic changes in the vessels of rheumatic patients in the third and fourth decades of life was mainly composed of fatty streaks; in older subjects raised lesions predominated.

Some variations in atherosclerosis depending on sex were noted in the patients with RHD. The area with atherosclerotic changes, excluding lipidosis in the aorta, was greater in males than in females. Especially large differences between the sexes were present in the degree of atherosclerosis in the coronary arteries. In the abdominal aorta the area with raised lesions in the third decade of life occupied 2.7% in males and 2.6% in females; in the fourth decade, 8.7% and 7.5%; in the fifth decade, 22.5% and 24.3%; in the sixth, 34% and 36.2%, and in the seventh, 51.9% and 43.8% of the intimal surface, respectively. In the LAD coronary artery raised lesions in the third decade of life occupied 1.7% in males and 0.9% in females; in the fourth, 8.9% and 3.0%;

in the fifth, 17.7% and 10.8%; in the sixth, 18.8% and 21.0%; and in the seventh, 37.8% and 24.3% of the intimal surface, respectively.

Stenosis of the coronary arteries by 50% or more was rare in patients with RHD. It was present in males only in the sixth and seventh decades of life and then only in four of 64 cases. In females such stenoses were present only in the seventh decade of life and only in four cases.

COMPARISON OF ATHEROSCLEROTIC STAGES IN PATIENTS WITH RHD AND IN EHI

In both groups in the third decade of life males showed various atherosclerotic changes in the aorta in all cases. In females in both groups there were isolated cases without any changes in the thoracic aorta.

In EHI the changes in the aorta were often restricted to lipidosis; in males the differences between the groups were statistically significant in nearly all decades of life and in respect to age-standardized (20–69 years) indices of the frequency of affected vessels. In females the differences between the groups in each decade of life were less significant, but were statistically significant when compared by age-standardized indices (Table 30). It is interesting that in the sixth decade of life in the thoracic aorta of healthy males and in the abdominal aorta of healthy females, Stage 1 atherosclerosis (i.e., only lipidosis) was found more frequently, in 17.2 and 9.4% of cases, respectively. In patients with RHD in this decade of life there were more severe atherosclerotic changes in the aorta in all observations.

EHI often showed fatty streaks in the aorta while in patients with RHD a combination of lipidosis and fibrous plaques was often noted. The differences between the groups were statistically significant in individual decades of life and according to age-standardized indices. More severe atherosclerotic changes, i.e., complicated lesions and calcification, in the abdominal aorta were also frequently seen in patients with RHD. In the thoracic aorta of females there were no differences between the groups, but in males these changes were noted more frequently in EHI (Table 30). Coronary arteries without any atherosclerotic changes were observed quite frequently in both groups. The differences between the groups in the frequency of such arteries in individual decades of life were usually neither statistically significant nor unidirectional. On the basis of the age-standardized index for the left circumflex coronary artery, arteries without changes were most often present in males and females with RHD, and in essentially healthy females; a similar situation was found with regard to the right coronary artery (Table 31).

Coronary arteries with only fatty streaks in males and females were usually seen more frequently in healthy people than in patients with RHD. However,

Table 30. Age-standardized (20–69 years) Indices of Prevalence of Atherosclerotic Changes in EHI (1) and RHD Patients (2)

Vessels	Group	Lipidosis only		Lipidosis and fibrous plaques		Complicated lesions and calcification	
		M	F	M	F	M	F
ThA	1	44.3	46.4	41.1	41.8	12.4	11.5
	2	22.2*	37.0*	65.6*	48.6*	8.2*	12.7
AA	1	29.9	35.0	41.3	43.5	19.0	21.5
	2	10.7*	20.4*	54.6*	51.3*	34.9*	28.3*
RCA	1	28.7	39.2	47.1	43.4	13.1	9.8
	2	21.6*	31.7*	53.4*	46.7	14.7	7.0
LCCA	1	25.9	40.2	49.6	36.3	8.6	4.8
	2	23.5	27.1*	49.4	44.6*	7.9	5.6
LADCA	1	16.8	28.5	62.1	52.7	17.2	12.1
	2	13.8*	26.3	60.5	56.3	20.9	10.4

ThA, thoracic aorta; AA, abdominal aorta; RCA, right coronary artery; LCCA, left circumflex coronary artery; LADCA, left anterior descending coronary artery.
* Differences statistically significant ($p \leqslant 0.05$). Prevalence given as percentage of cases.

Table 31. Age-standardized (20–69 years) Indices of Percentage of Coronary Arteries without Changes in EHI (1) and RHD Patients (2)

Sex	Group	Right coronary artery	Left circumflex coronary artery	Left anterior descending coronary artery
Males	1	11.2	15.9	3.9
	2	10.2	19.1*	4.8
Females	1	18.1	18.2	6.6
	2	11.4*	22.7*	7.2

* Differences statistically significant ($p \leqslant 0.05$).

the differences between the groups in individual decades of life were as a rule not statistically significant; in some of the comparisons age-standardized indices showed significant differences between the groups (Table 30).

Differences between the groups in the frequency of fatty streaks and fibrous plaques in the coronary arteries in individual decades of life were not marked, but the changes were somewhat more frequent in patients with RHD. The differences in age-standardized indices were significant in the right coronary artery in males and in the left circumflex coronary artery in females. Coronary arteries with complicated lesions and calcification were present in both groups with more or less the same frequency. Comparisons of the groups in individual decades of life and in age-standardized indices did not reveal significant differences (Table 30).

COMPARISONS OF ATHEROSCLEROTIC AREAS IN EHI AND RHD PATIENTS

The total area with atherosclerotic changes in both parts of the aorta in males and females was usually greater in patients with RHD than in healthy people (Fig. 23). The differences observed were statistically significant in the thoracic aorta for males in the third, fifth, and sixth decades of life, and for females, in the fourth, fifth, and sixth decades of life; in the abdominal aorta for males in the fourth and sixth, and for females in the third through sixth decades of life. The rise in the total area with atherosclerotic changes in patients with RHD in both parts of the aorta was due to the greater extent of fatty streaks and especially fibrous plaques in these patients as compared with healthy people.

In the coronary arteries the total area with atherosclerotic change was the same in both groups or slightly less in patients with RHD than in healthy people (Fig. 23). The differences were statistically significant for the left anterior descending coronary artery in males in the third and sixth decades of life, and in females in the third, fourth, and seventh decades of life and for the left circumflex coronary artery only in females in the third decade of life. The observed differences were mainly due to the varying extent of fibrous plaques in the two groups.

The total area with atherosclerotic changes in patients dying from the various complications of atherosclerosis was almost always considerably higher than in patients suffering from RHD and in healthy people. The differences in patients dying from the various complications of atherosclerosis were mainly due to the great extent of atherosclerosis with raised lesions (fibrous plaques, complicated lesions, and calcification).

We now present data showing the areas with individual types of atherosclerotic changes in both groups. In both parts of the aorta the differences in the area with fatty streaks between the groups were not unidirectional. Therefore, they were rarely statistically significant, especially between the corresponding groups of females. The differences between the groups were also not statistically significant for the age-standardized indices of the area with lipidosis (Table 32).

The differences between the groups in the area with lipidosis in the coronary arteries were not great, but a clear tendency to a lower degree of lipidosis was present in patients with RHD. During a comparison of the groups in the indi-

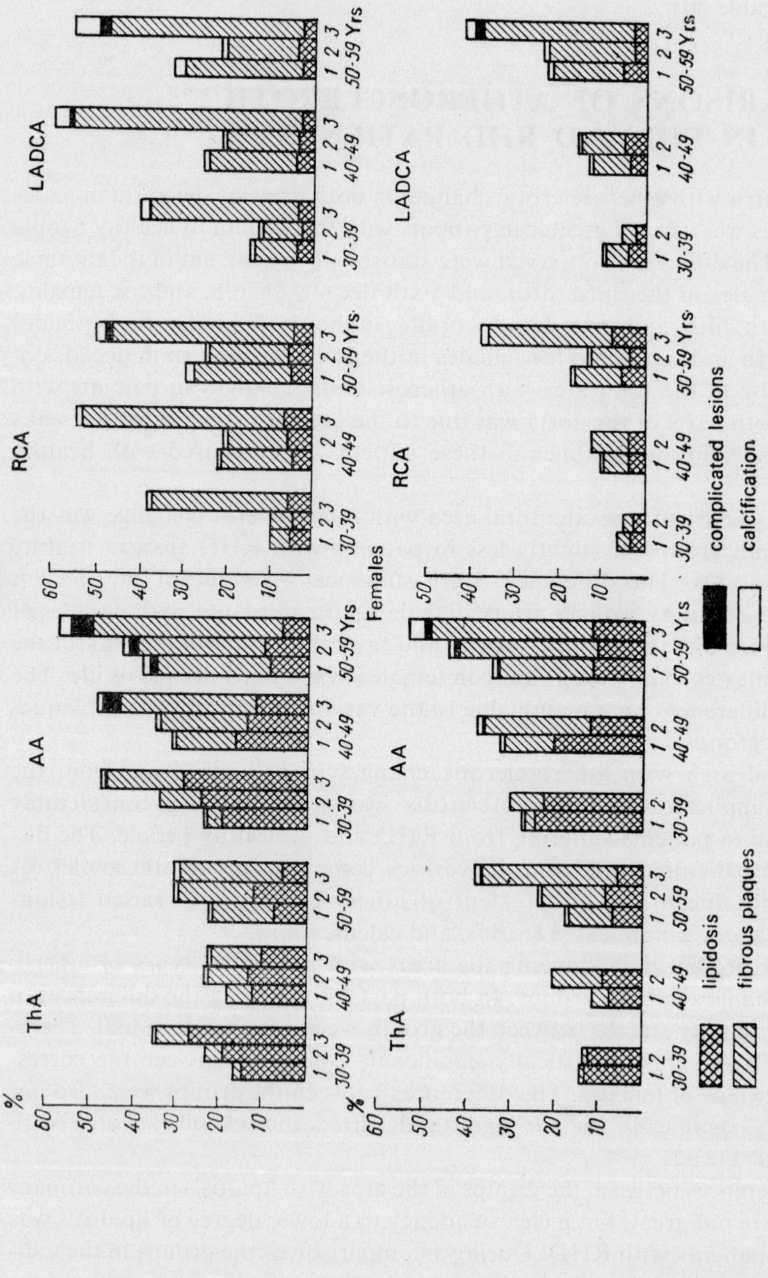

Figure 23. Characteristics of atherosclerotic changes in the aorta and coronary arteries of EHI (*1*), RHD patients (*2*), and patients dying from complications of atherosclerosis (*3*). ThA, thoracic aorta; AA, abdominal aorta; RCA, right coronary artery; LADCA, left anterior descending coronary artery. The ordinate shows the changed area as a percentage of the intimal surface of the vessel.

vidual decades of life this was noted in 19 of 30 comparisons ($p_{kz} > 0.05$). Age-standardized indices of the area with lipidosis in the coronary arteries also indicate a low degree of lipidosis in patients with RHD (Table 32).

Table 32. Age-standardized (20–69 years) Indices for Raised Lesions and Lipidosis in EHI (1) and RHD patients (2)

Type of change	Group	ThA	AA	RCA	LCCA	LADCA
Males						
Lipidosis	1	8.7	15.2	3.8	3.2	3.0
	2	8.7	16.0	3.8	2.8	2.3
Raised lesions	1	10.5	19.6	16.9	14.5	21.2
	2	11.6	24.6*	17.6	11.2*	17.0*
Females						
Lipidosis	1	9.7	17.2	2.9	3.7	3.6
	2	8.5	15.4	3.2	2.9	2.5*
Raised lesions	1	8.9	16.0	9.9	9.0	13.6
	2	12.7*	22.9*	8.6	6.7*	12.0

ThA, thoracic aorta; AA, abdominal aorta; RCA, right coronary artery; LCCA, left circumflex coronary artery; LADCA, left anterior descending coronary artery. Areas given as percentage of intimal surface of vessel.

* Differences statistically significant ($p \leqslant 0.05$).

The area occupied by fibrous plaques in the aorta was almost always greater (in 18 of 20 comparisons; $p_{kz} < 0.01$) in patients with RHD than in healthy people (Fig. 23). These differences between the groups according to the decade of life were statistically significant in 11 comparisons; age-standardized indices of the area with fibrous plaques were considerably greater for the group of patients with RHD.

In the coronary arteries the area occupied by fibrous plaques was usually smaller (in 20 of 30 comparisons; $p_{kz} = 0.05$). In patients with RHD, however, the differences between the groups in individual decades of life very rarely attained statistically significant indices (only in five comparisons). Age-standardized indices of the area with fibrous plaques in the coronary arteries were also less in a group of patients with RHD.

The extent of complicated lesions in the vessels was more or less the same in the groups.

The degree of calcification in the aorta of males and females was the same in the two groups. In the coronary arteries the area with calcification was significantly greater in essentially healthy males only in the sixth decade of life, and in essentially healthy females only in the seventh decade of life, compared with patients with RHD. In other decades of life there were no significant differences between the groups.

The area with raised lesions (fibrous plaques, complicated lesions, and calcification) in the aorta of males and females was always greater in patients with RHD than in healthy people. The differences between the groups were statistically significant in half of the comparisons of the groups in individual decades of life. The differences were also significant for the age-standardized indices for the abdominal aorta in males and females and the thoracic aorta in females only (Table 32). In all the coronary arteries the area with raised lesions was often somewhat less in patients with RHD than in healthy people; age-standardized indices of the area with raised lesions showed significant differences between the groups in the left circumflex coronary artery in males and females and in the left anterior descending coronary artery in males (Table 32).

Stenosis of the coronary arteries by 50% or more of the lumen was noted in the older age groups in patients with RHD. In healthy people the stenoses appeared in the fifth decade of life. In patients with RHD the changes appeared one (in males) or two (in females) decades later. In addition, the frequency of cases with stenosis of the coronary arteries was usually higher in the group of healthy people than in the group of patients with RHD. In healthy males 50 to 59 years old stenoses were present in 8.5% of cases, but in patients with RHD in only 1.9% ($p \leqslant 0.01$); in females of 60 to 69 years the stenoses were present in 16.5 and 8.7% of cases, respectively ($p \leqslant 0.05$).

The data comparing the areas occupied by the various types of atherosclerotic change demonstrate the following: (1) in both parts of the aorta atherosclerosis develops more rapidly in patients with RHD than in the healthy; the total area with atherosclerotic changes and the area with raised lesions were as a rule larger in patients with RHD than in a group of healthy people. (2) In the coronary arteries there was a definite tendency toward a lower degree of atherosclerosis in patients with RHD than in healthy people; the total area with atherosclerotic changes and the area with raised lesions were often less in RHD; the atherosclerotic index was more or less the same in the groups, or lower in the RHD group. (3) In both parts of the aorta the maximum differences between the groups were noted in the area occupied by fibrous plaques; the differences in other types of atherosclerotic lesions were usually not significant but at the same time not multidirectional.

In most cases atherosclerotic changes in patients with RHD did not show any special features during macroscopic study of the vessels. Only in a small number of cases were special characteristics of the atherosclerotic process noted; these were mostly in the abdominal aorta. The features tended to a diffuse type of intimal lesion. The fibrous plaques were thick, smooth, white in color, usually without clear-cut boundaries, and often fused together; the surface of the plaques was slightly puckered.

Histological and histochemical studies of the aorta (100 cases) and the coronary arteries (40 cases) in most cases revealed focal and, on rare occasions, diffuse accumulation of acid mucopolysaccharides in the form of hyaluronic acid and chondroitin sulfates in the sclerosed intima and in the fibrous covering of the plaques; even in the media there was an uneven accumulation of acid mucopolysaccharides. The changes observed were localized and were mostly seen in the region of atherosclerotic plaques. They were rarely observed beyond their boundaries.

There was often sclerosis in the adventitia of the vessels studied with infiltration of a small number of lymphoid cells (Fig. 24), which sometimes extended along the course of the small vessels in the outer third of the media. The most marked sclerotic changes were usually found around the vasa vasorum of the aorta. It should be emphasized that the above changes were usually observed in areas of the vessels with atherosclerotic changes in the intima.

We did not observe rheumatic nodules in the wall of the aorta or coronary arteries in a single case. In one case, in a thoracic aorta there were signs of an old, severe aortitis with a primary lesion in the media and adventitia; we found extensive destruction of the elastic fibers, sclerosis and infiltration of lymphoid cells (Fig. 25).

During histological examination of the aorta in subjects dying from RHD we also noted changes indicating participation of a mural thrombus in the development of atherosclerotic plaques; thrombotic masses were present on the surface of the plaques and throughout their depth (Fig. 26).

The lipid content of atherosclerotic plaques in RHD is diverse in nature, although plaques with a large amount of lipids and especially those with atheromatous degeneration are rarely seen.

The data indicate that in both parts of the aorta atherosclerotic changes develop at more rapid rates in those with RHD than in healthy people. However, there were no differences between these groups in the degree of atherosclerosis in the coronary arteries. On the contrary, the extent of atherosclerotic changes was less in patients with RHD. Our data are in agreement with the findings of Wang and Hu (1957) who also noted intense development of atherosclerosis in the aorta without intensification of this process in the coronary arteries.

The conflicting opinions concerning the significance of RHD in the development of atherosclerosis partly result from the subjective factors in the assessment of the degree of atherosclerosis in autopsy forms and the difficulty of analyzing autopsy materials for this purpose. The intensifying effect of RHD on the development of atherosclerosis is to some degree related to the various microscopic changes in the vessels in patients with RHD. But it must be noted that specific rheumatic changes were usually demonstrable only in smaller vessels (Talalaev, 1929; Skvortsov, 1938; Strukov, 1961; Mitin, 1966; Strukov and Beglaryan, 1963). In large arteries and the aorta rheumatic nodules are rarely noted, although nonspecific changes can frequently be seen in these vessels. In this respect the findings of Mikhailov (1966) are of

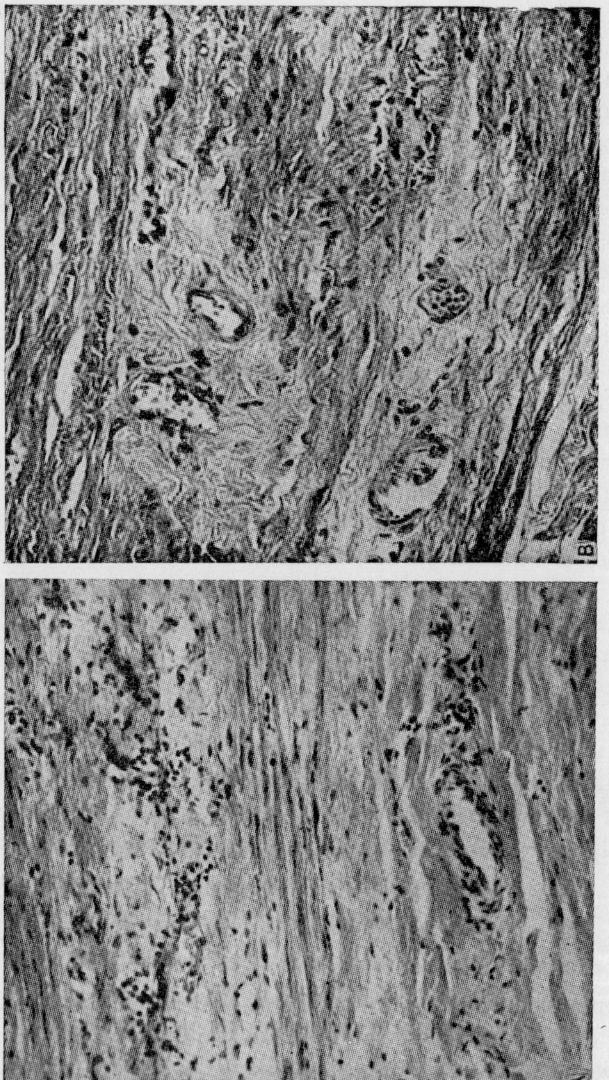

Figure 24. (*A*), Infiltration of a small number of lymphoid cells and perivascular sclerosis; (*B*), the changes in the adventitia and neighboring areas of the media in the aorta. Magnification: *A* × 205, *B* × 165. Staining, hematoxylin and eosin.

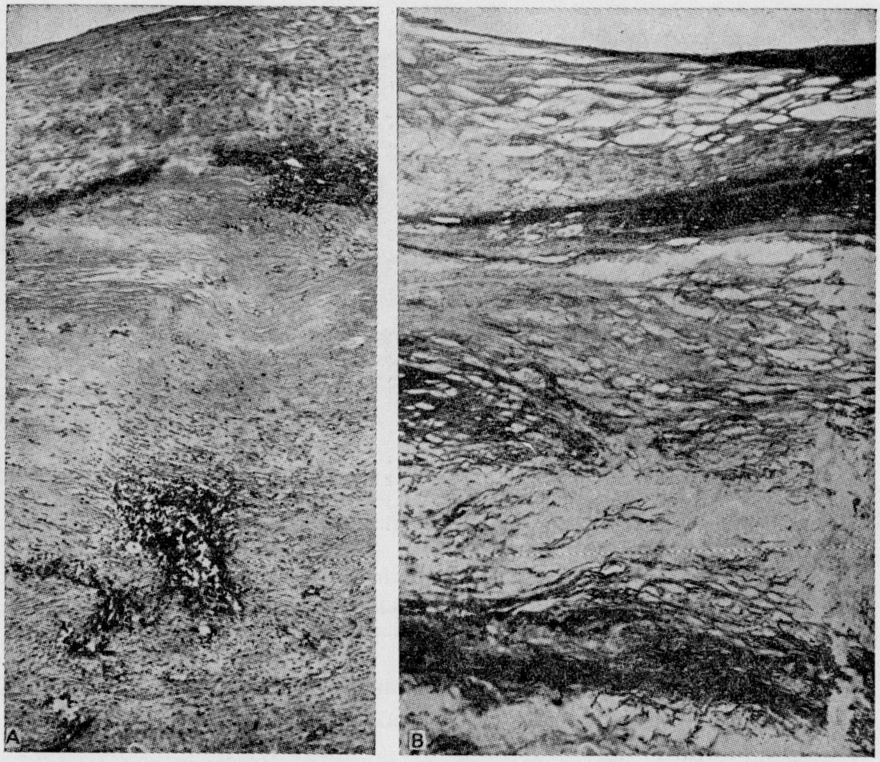

Figure 25. Severe sclerosis of aortic wall with large infiltration of lymphoid cells (*A*) and destruction of elastic structures (*B*). Magnification, *A* × 65; *B* × 65. Staining, *A*, hematoxylin-eosin; *B*, fuchsin.

importance. In the aorta of children under age 16 he frequently observed changes in the elastic laminae, fatty and lymphatic infiltrations in the intima, and, in only one case of 38, the formation of rheumatic nodules.

In the course of microscopic examination of 100 aortas and 40 coronary arteries we did not observe rheumatic nodules in the walls of these vessels in a single case; various nonspecific changes (sclerosis of the adventitia, infiltrations of lymphoid cells in the adventitia and the outer third of the media, mucoidal edema of sclerosed intima, and fibrous coverings of the plaques) were found frequently.

These changes were most common in the aorta. This suggests that nonspecific changes in the aortic wall precede the rapid development of atherosclerosis in the aorta in RHD. This opinion is shared by Mitin (1966).

In the course of microscopic examination of the aorta we frequently noted considerable amounts of proteinaceous masses and collections of fine layers of fibrin on the surface of the plaques and throughout their depth. This in-

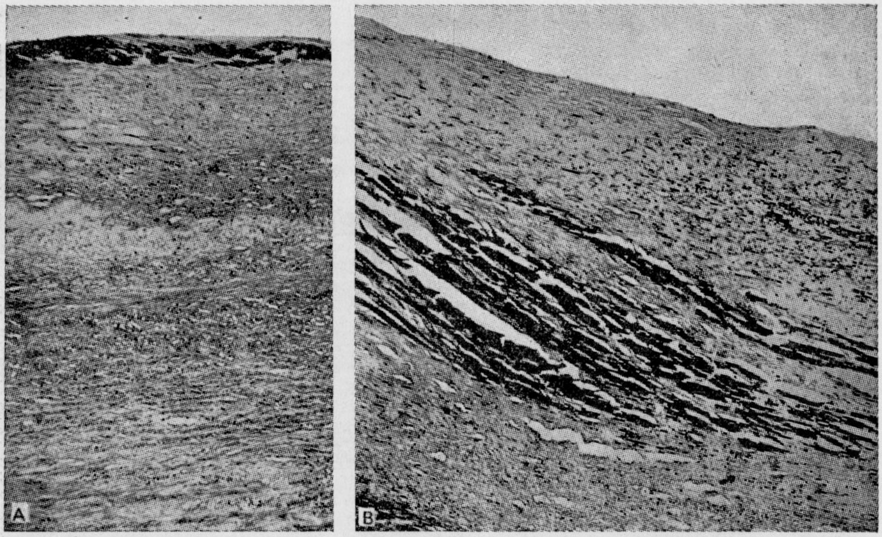

Figure 26. Accumulation of proteinaceous (fibrinous) masses on the surface (*A*) and throughout the depth (*B*) of atherosclerotic plaques in the aorta. Magnification × 63. Masson stain.

dicates the possible contribution of the coagulation system to the accelerated development of atherosclerosis in the aorta in certain stages of RHD (Syurin, 1966; Grigor'eva, 1967).

It is probable that the chronic venous congestion of the aortic wall, observed in conjunction with valvular diseases of the heart, also has some significance for the development of atherosclerosis in the aorta of patients with RHD.

It is interesting that in RHD intense development of atherosclerosis was observed only in the aorta. In the coronary arteries, on the other hand, we noted a tendency toward less atherosclerosis than in healthy people. This indicates that the development of atherosclerosis in different parts of the arterial system has its own characteristics, resulting from the structure and metabolism of different vessels, the organ's specific circulation, and possibly other factors. These conditions affect the degree of atherosclerosis differently in different arteries in patients with RHD, in other patients, and in healthy people.

It is possible that hypoxia is one of the factors that contributes to the slow development of atherosclerosis in the coronary arteries in RHD. Hypoxia produces an increase in the coronary circulation and dilatation of the coronary vessels. In addition, in patients with rheumatic heart disease there are often changes in lipid metabolism opposite to those found in patients with atherosclerosis, and this too may be responsible for the slow development of atherosclerosis in the coronary arteries in RHD (Mikunis, 1963; Petrovskii *et al.*, 1972). It should also be noted that patients with RHD have fewer non-specific changes in the coronary arteries than in the aorta. The data presented partly explain the varying degrees of atherosclerosis in the aorta and coronary arteries in patients with RHD.

7

Atherosclerosis and Chronic Lung Diseases

Chronic nonspecific inflammatory lung diseases include chronic bronchitis, diffuse membranous pneumosclerosis, chronic obstructive pulmonary disease (COPD), and bronchiectasis. Right ventricular hypertrophy, often with dilatation (cor pulmonale), is a characteristic sign of the cases belonging to this group. Not much information is available in the literature on the features of the development of atherosclerosis in patients with COPD.

Most investigators have concluded that the development of atherosclerosis in patients with COPD is slower than in other patients (Wang and Hu, 1957; Smolenskii, 1960b, 1964; Shalevich and Sarankin, 1962; Damir and Sarankin, 1963; Roguski *et al.*, 1964; Kolomoiskaya, 1964; Shapiro, 1966; Alikhanova, 1968). Smolenskii (1960b) found that 49 patients dying from COPD did not show atherosclerosis at autopsy; 28 patients showed mild or moderate atherosclerosis, and 9 patients showed marked atherosclerosis but were without thrombonecrotic complications or marked clinical manifestations. In only 11 patients were severe forms of atherosclerosis observed. Smolenskii stressed that the pulmonary processes associated with an infection of the bronchial tree to a great extent inhibited atherosclerosis. The incidence of pronounced atherosclerosis in patients with suppurative bronchitis and infective bronchiectasis was half that of patients without suppurative infection of the respiratory tract.

Kolomoiskaya (1964) analyzed 206 autopsy forms and case histories of subjects dying from COPD. The cases were subdivided into four groups according to the degree of atherosclerosis. A very severe degree of atherosclerosis was found in only 11 cases, i.e., in 5.6%. In most cases (80.6%) the lesions were of a mild degree.

Myocardial infarction in patients with COPD was less common than in other patients, which is also related to the low degree of atherosclerosis of the coronary arteries in these patients (Zlochevskii, 1964; Nonkin *et al.*,

1964; Samad and Noehren, 1965; Shapiro, 1966; Simagina *et al.*, 1968).

There are also reports in the literature that marked atherosclerosis is very common in COPD. Sipovskii and Vlasova (1961), in a study of pathological material collected from 1954 through 1958 in Leningrad, found atherosclerosis in 51.6% of cases of chronic nonspecific diseases of the lungs. However, the authors give no data showing the degree of atherosclerosis in these cases. Andrushchenko (1964), Baizakova (1967), and others have noted the frequent presence of atherosclerosis in patients with COPD. On the basis of an analysis of 219 autopsy forms of those dying from COPD Panfilov and Rusakov (1966) concluded that chronic pulmonary diseases do not inhibit the development of atherosclerosis. After studying the clinical signs of atherosclerosis in lung diseases associated with the development of cor pulmonale, Roguski *et al.* (1964) supported this view. These authors conclude that lung diseases neither retard nor favor the development of atherosclerosis.

There are few reports showing the rates of development of atherosclerotic changes in specific arteries in patients with COPD. Kolomoiskaya (1964) noted that in these patients atherosclerotic changes were more pronounced in the aorta than in the coronary arteries; atherosclerosis was least pronounced in the cerebral vessels. Wang and Hu (1957) found that in chronic lung diseases atherosclerosis develops more slowly in the coronary arteries than in the aorta.

Some authors (Tomas, 1958; Mikhnev *et al.*, 1961) incorrectly considered frequent pains in the precordial region and certain changes in the ECG in patients with COPD as evidence for coronary atherosclerosis. This error has been pointed out by Smolenskii (1960b), Kolomoiskaya (1964), Shapiro (1966), and others.

Most authors relate the inhibitory effect of chronic pneumonia on the development of atherosclerosis to a series of complex phenomena characterizing this disease. In patients with COPD there is rarely any rise in arterial blood pressure; on the contrary, hypotension frequently occurs (Smolenskii, 1960b; Kolomoiskaya, 1964; Shapiro, 1966; Simagina *et al.*, 1968). Interesting data are provided by Shalovich and Sarankin (1962), who failed to observe any appreciable difference in the prevalence of atherosclerosis in the coronary arteries of patients who died from COPD coupled with hypertension (13 cases) and the main group of patients with pulmonary diseases. These data probably indicate that the atherogenic effect of hypertension in those patients is neutralized by other factors showing inhibitory effect on the development of atherosclerosis. To some extent this occurs because the rise in arterial hypertension in patients with COPD is often present for only a short period (Tomas, 1958).

Many authors think that disorders of lipid metabolism contribute to the slow development of atherosclerosis in patients with COPD (Smolenskii, 1960b; Roguski *et al.*, 1964; Baizakova, 1967; Mutina, 1968). The characteristic changes in chronic pneumonia include a tendency to hypocholesterolemia, a rise in the level of β-lipoproteins, a fall in the level of α-lipoproteins, and several other disorders of lipid metabolism.

According to some researchers, the observed metabolic disorders and a tendency to hypotension are due to chronic drug addiction and hypoxia (Smolenskii, 1960a; Sarankin, 1963; Kolomoiskaya, 1964).

The significance of hypoxia in the development of atherosclerotic changes has not yet been determined. Some studies indicate that there is an intensification of atherosclerotic changes in hypoxia (Kipshidze, 1959; Altland and Higman, 1960; Mikhnev *et al.*, 1961; Kyeldsen *et al.*, 1968). Others hold the opposite view and think that hypoxia has an inhibitory effect (Smolenskii, 1960a; Kolomoiskaya, 1964). It is probable that hypoxia does not act in a uniform manner in all the arteries. Its most significant effect is on the development of atherosclerosis in the coronary arteries. Hypoxia may cause an increase in the coronary circulation with dilatation of the coronary arteries and the intense development of intercoronary anastomoses (Berezhnitskii, 1962; Nonkin *et al.*, 1964; Van Liere and Stickney, 1967). It is possible that the inhibitory effect of hypoxia is seen only in the presence of certain conditions, for example, in conjunction with hypocholesterolemia and hypotension. However, according to the experimental data of Kipshidze (1959), hypoxia in rabbits in conjunction with hypercholesterolemia leads to more marked development of experimental lipidosis in the aorta and coronary arteries than in control groups.

The effect of hypoxia on the development of coronary atherosclerosis is due not only to a change in the coronary hemodynamics but also to other conditions. In particular, hypoxia affects the lipolytic activity of the various organs and vascular walls (Dixon, 1961; Uspenskii and Chzhou-Su, 1963). Hypoxia frequently lowers the arterial pressure and causes adrenal insufficiency (Armstrong and Heim, 1938) and decreases the action of the coagulation system (Myasnikov, 1965; Van Liere and Stickney, 1963).

It has been demonstrated that the lungs have an active role in lipid metabolism. In a number of studies (Hine, 1935; Vilkovysskii and Zakhar'in, 1959; Mosinger *et al.*, 1964; Babushkina, 1966; Leites, 1967) it has been shown that if surplus fat enters the lungs, part of it is retained and later destroyed. The degradation of fat is probably due to the activity of lipoprotein lipase and its cofactor heparin, which are present in high concentration in the lungs (Voinova, 1967). It may be that this system is altered to a considerable extent in chronic pulmonary diseases, and hypocholesterolemia and other disorders of lipid metabolism to some extent result from disorders in the lipid metabolism of the lungs.

Besides the above factors, some investigators attribute the inhibitory effect of COPD on the development of atherosclerosis to a change in the coagulation system. But the data showing changes in the coagulation process in

COPD are contradictory. In such patients some workers noted a fall in the activity of the coagulation process (Il'yasov, 1966; Yushina, 1967); others found a fall in the activity of the anticoagulation process (Syurin, 1966; Evdokimov, 1968). Probably the coagulation process of the blood may change depending on the stage of the disease (Yushina, 1967). This would explain the contradictions in the available data. Similarly the other factors that often accompany COPD, like emaciation and adrenal failure, may have some effect on the development of atherosclerosis. It is necessary to emphasize that all these factors do not operate in isolation from each other but, as a rule, act simultaneously, i.e., various factors in combination affect the development of atherosclerosis. Since the available data describing the course of the atherosclerotic process in patients with COPD are not sufficient we conducted a morphometric study of atherosclerosis in 329 such cases (Table 33). All cases with a combination of several other diseases were excluded from the analysis.

Table 33. Age and Sex Distribution of COPD Cases

Age in years	30–39	40–49	50–59	60–69	70–79	Total
Males	20	31	51	76	40	218
Females	—	14	25	43	29	111

The prevalence, and similarly the area with atherosclerotic changes and the area with raised lesions, increased with the age of the patients. In the fourth decade of life in males and in the fifth decade of life in females there were fatty streaks and fibrous plaques in the aorta and coronary arteries in most cases. In the eighth decade of life complicated lesions and calcification were present in most cases. The latter were noted in the abdominal aorta in 83% of the males and in 89.7% of the females; and in the left anterior descending coronary artery in 62.5% and 57.1% of the cases, respectively.

Some sex variations in the degree of atherosclerosis were noted in the patients with COPD. In most comparisons the area with atherosclerotic changes (except the areas with fatty streaks) was somewhat larger in males than in females (Table 34).

Stenosis of the coronary arteries by 50% or more was noted in patients with COPD after the sixth decade of life and was observed somewhat more frequently in males than in females; age-standardized (50–79) indices of the frequency of this stenosis were 13.9% and 8.7%, respectively ($p \leqslant 0.05$).

Table 34. Area with Atherosclerotic Changes in COPD Patients

Age in years	Values*	Abdominal aorta					Left anterior descending coronary artery				
		TA	F	FbPl	Co	Ca	TA	F	FbPl	Co	Ca
Males											
40–49	M	25.5	9.9	15.0	0.1	0.3	11.5	1.8	9.1	0	0.6
	SE	1.9	1.3	1.9	0.7	0.2	1.9	0.4	1.5	0	0.5
50–59	M	37.3	3.6	29.4	0.8	3.4	23.8	1.5	19.4	0.06	2.6
	SE	2.8	0.3	9.5	0.3	1.2	2.2	0.2	1.6	0.04	0.8
60–69	M	53.8	2.7	41.2	3.0	6.9	36.0	1.5	26.9	0.2	7.4
	SE	1.7	0.2	1.5	0.3	0.8	1.9	0.1	1.6	0.1	1.5
70–79	M	58.0	3.4	45.1	3.6	5.9	47.8	2.5	38.2	0.5	6.6
	SE	3.2	0.6	2.8	0.7	1.7	3.8	0.4	2.8	0.3	1.1
Females											
40–49	M	20.3	8.9	10.8	6.2	0.4	12.2	2.0	10.2	0.0	0.0
	SE	5.5	1.8	4.6	0.6	0.08	3.2	0.5	2.6	0	0
50–59	M	29.5	8.6	19.5	0.2	1.2	20.5	2.4	13.7	0.04	4.3
	SE	2.8	1.8	2.9	0.1	0.8	3.8	0.5	3.3	0	2.5
60–69	M	45.2	3.6	37.7	0.9	3.0	31.6	2.0	25.9	0	3.7
	SE	3.0	0.5	2.6	0.3	0.5	2.5	0.3	2.4	0	0.7
70–79	M	55.7	3.1	44.8	2.0	5.8	40.0	2.7	29.1	0.07	8.1
	SE	3.9	0.3	3.4	1.1	1.1	4.1	0.5	3.3	0.3	3.0

* M, mean; SE, standard error; TA, total area with atherosclerotic changes; F, fatty streaks; FbPl, fibrous plaques; Co, complicated lesions; Ca, calcification. Area given as percentage of intimal surface of vessels.

ATHEROSCLEROTIC FREQUENCY IN EHI AND COPD PATIENTS

In the aorta there were various atherosclerotic changes in all cases in both the groups. The maximal differences in the frequency of atherosclerotic changes in the aorta (particularly in the descending thoracic aorta) were noted when comparing the corresponding groups of males. In both parts of the aorta in essentially healthy males only fatty streaks were often found. In patients with COPD there were fibrous plaques in combination with lipidosis (thoracic aorta) or more severe changes, especially complicated lesions and calcification in both parts of the aorta (Table 35). The frequency of calcification in the aorta (without considering complicated lesions) was likewise more frequent in patients with COPD. In the abdominal aorta of healthy males 40 to 79 years of age, calcification was present in 48.7% of the cases; in patients

Table 35. Age-standardized (males 30–79, females 40–79 years) Indices of Atherosclerotic Changes in EHI (1) and COPD Patients (2)

Type of change	Groups	ThA	AA	RCA	LCCA	LADCA
Males						
No change	1	—	—	5.2	7.8	1.2
	2	—	—	10.1*	15.7*	6.9*
Lipidosis only	1	27.2	14.0	19.3	18.9	10.1
	2	10.0*	10.5	19.8	17.6	12.3
Lipidosis & fibrous plaques	1	46.6	40.1	52.9	57.7	60.0
	2	58.5*	40.6	47.6	48.5*	48.4*
Complicated lesions & calcification	1	24.8	45.9	22.5	15.5	28.7
	2	30.7*	48.1	22.6	18.2	32.4
Females						
No change	1	—	—	6.3	6.1	1.8
	2	—	—	4.8	5.2	4.9
Lipidosis only	1	14.2	9.2	23.8	25.2	14.1
	2	15.5	7.7	13.9*	20.5	5.3*
Lipidosis & fibrous plaques	1	50.7	45.3	48.7	53.7	53.4
	2	52.2	42.7	66.9*	59.7	56.6
Complicated lesions & calcification	1	32.3	46.2	20.5	15.0	30.8
	2	32.3	48.1	16.6	14.6	33.1

ThA, thoracic aorta; AA, abdominal aorta; RCA, right coronary artery; LCCA, left circumflex coronary artery; LADCA, left anterior descending coronary artery.

* Differences statistically significant ($p \leqslant 0.05$). Frequency expressed as percentage of intimal surface of vessels.

with COPD, in 53.8%; in females, in 42.9% and 45.1% of the cases, respectively (age-standardized indices). The differences in the frequency of atherosclerotic lesions in both parts of the aorta between the two groups of females were not significant (Table 35).

Coronary arteries without any atherosclerotic changes were observed in subjects of both groups up to 70 years of age. Unaffected arteries were observed more frequently in males with COPD than in healthy people; the differences between the corresponding groups of females were not significant.

There were no significant differences in the frequency of very mild (lipidosis) and very severe (complicated lesions and calcification) lesions between the two groups of males. However, there were differences in the frequency of fibrous plaques in combination with lipidosis. Such coronary arteries were seen more frequently in EHI. Between the corresponding groups of females there were sometimes no significant differences in the frequency of changes in the coronary arteries. Nevertheless, in healthy females there were frequently coronary arteries with lipidosis only, and the patients with COPD showed lipidosis with fibrous plaques. There were no significant differences between the groups in the frequency of very severe changes (complicated lesions and calcification). An analysis of the frequency of cases with calcification of the coronary arteries (independent of the presence of complicated lesions) failed to reveal any significant differences between the groups although, as with the aorta, calcification was more frequent in patients with COPD.

ATHEROSCLEROTIC AREAS IN EHI AND COPD PATIENTS

The total area with atherosclerotic changes, and similarly the area with raised lesions in the thoracic aorta, were usually more extensive in patients with COPD (Fig. 27); the differences between the groups were statistically significant in males in most decades of life, in females in the sixth decade of life. Considerable differences in the degree of these changes in the abdominal aorta in any particular direction were not noted in individual decades, particularly in the areas with raised lesions; similarly no significant differences were noted in the age-standardized indices of the areas with raised lesions.

The total area of atherosclerotic changes, and similarly the total area of raised lesions, in the coronary arteries of males and females with COPD was smaller than in healthy people (Fig. 27). The differences between the corresponding groups of males were statistically significant in practically all decades of life and in age-standardized indices; between the two groups of females the differences were usually not significant, but the same tendency was noted (Table 36).

The atherosclerotic index, calculated on the basis of the area and degree of

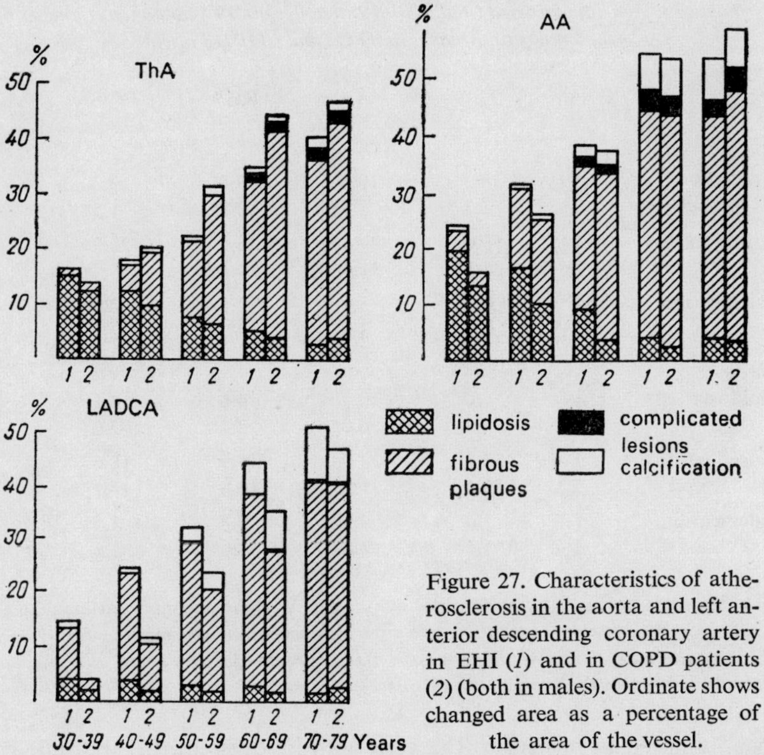

Figure 27. Characteristics of atherosclerosis in the aorta and left anterior descending coronary artery in EHI (*1*) and in COPD patients (*2*) (both in males). Ordinate shows changed area as a percentage of the area of the vessel.

severity of various types of atherosclerotic changes, shows the same characteristics for the patients with COPD as the data for the total area with atherosclerotic lesions and the area with raised lesions. The atherosclerotic index for the thoracic aorta was always higher in patients with COPD than in EHI, and was close to that in subjects dying from atherosclerosis. Even when the differences between the groups were significant in males, they were not high in the groups of females. The index for abdominal aorta was the same in both groups; in females with COPD the value was somewhat lower. The index for the coronary arteries was as a rule lower in patients with COPD, and the differences were often significant (Fig. 28).

The atherosclerotic index for the vessels of subjects dying from the various complications of atherosclerosis was always much higher than in a group of patients with COPD and in a group of healthy people (Fig. 28).

An analysis of the areas occupied by individual types of atherosclerotic change shows certain characteristics of the atherosclerotic process in the patients with COPD. In both parts of the aorta the area with fatty streaks in the coronary arteries of patients with COPD was as a rule smaller than in healthy subjects. The area with lipidosis was smaller in 42 of 45 comparisons between the groups ($p_{kz} < 0.01$). Major differences between the groups were

Table 36. Age-standardized (males 30–79, females 40–79 years of age) Indices of Atherosclerotic Areas in EHI (1) and COPD Patients (2)

Type of changes	Groups	ThA	AA	RCA	LCCA	LADCA
Males						
Lipidosis	1	8.3	10.6	3.8	3.3	2.8
	2	7.3	6.5*	2.2*	1.5*	1.8*
Raised lesions	1	18.0	29.4	26.0	22.9	30.6
	2	24.1*	31.4	20.4*	16.7*	22.7*
Calcification	1	0.7	3.1	2.1	2.0	3.7
	2	0.9	3.3	2.9	2.1	3.5
Females						
Lipidosis	1	6.0	10.7	4.6	4.1	3.6
	2	5.3	6.0*	2.7*	2.2*	2.3*
Raised lesions	1	22.3	33.0	18.9	18.6	26.2
	2	25.1	31.8	16.8	15.1*	23.8
Calcification	1	1.0	3.5	1.5	1.4	3.4
	2	1.1	2.8	1.0	1.6	4.0

ThA, thoracic aorta; AA, abdominal aorta; RCA, right coronary artery; LCCA, left circumflex coronary artery; LADCA, left anterior descending coronary artery.

* Differences statistically significant ($p \leqslant 0.05$). Diseased areas given as a percentage of the intimal surface of the vessels.

especially noted in respect to the area with lipidosis in the abdominal aorta and in the coronary arteries; the differences between the groups were statistically significant in more than two-thirds of the comparisons by individual decades of life and in age-standardized indices (Table 36).

In males and females with COPD fibrous plaques in the thoracic aorta always occupied a larger area than in healthy people; in males these differences were greater and often statistically significant. In the abdominal aorta the area with fibrous plaques was basically the same in both groups.

In the coronary arteries the area with fibrous plaques was almost always smaller in patients with COPD than in healthy people (Fig. 27); the differences were more marked between the groups of males than between the groups of females.

The differences between the groups in the area of complicated lesions were insignificant and in no particular direction; in more than half of the comparisons no differences between the groups in the area of complicated lesions were noticed.

The area with calcification increased with age in both groups. The differences between the groups were neither in the same direction nor statistically significant when compared by individual decades of life or on the basis of age-standardized indices (Table 36).

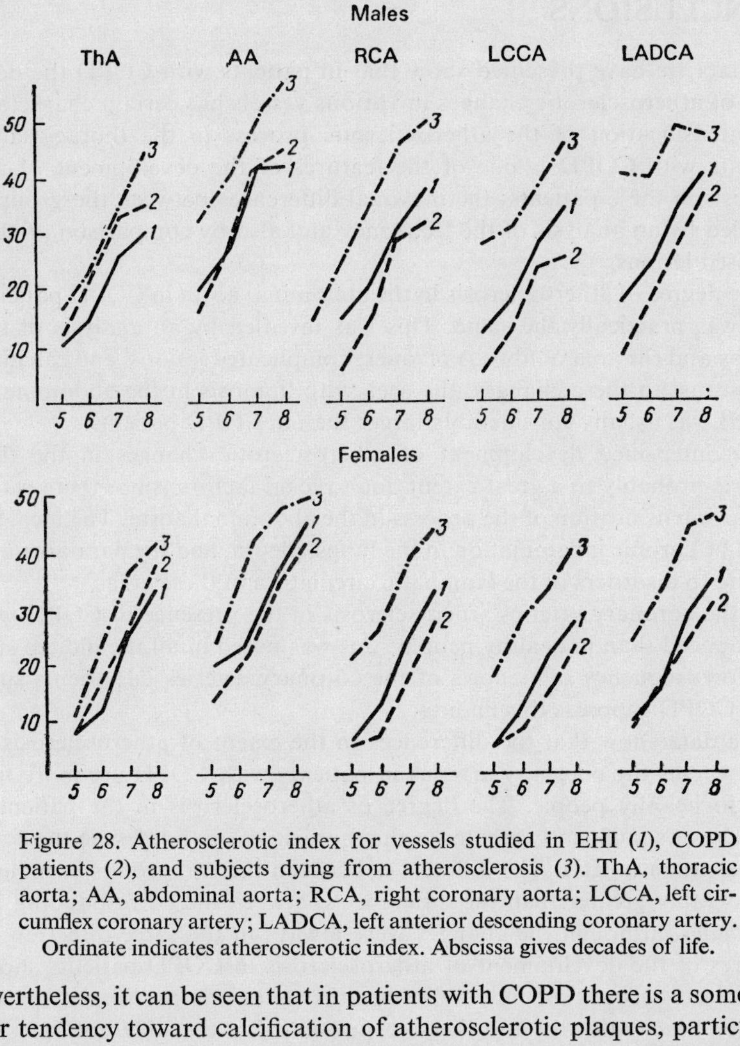

Figure 28. Atherosclerotic index for vessels studied in EHI (*1*), COPD patients (*2*), and subjects dying from atherosclerosis (*3*). ThA, thoracic aorta; AA, abdominal aorta; RCA, right coronary aorta; LCCA, left circumflex coronary artery; LADCA, left anterior descending coronary artery. Ordinate indicates atherosclerotic index. Abscissa gives decades of life.

Nevertheless, it can be seen that in patients with COPD there is a somewhat greater tendency toward calcification of atherosclerotic plaques, particularly in the coronary arteries of males. The absence of significant differences between the groups in the area of calcification supports this, although the area with fibrous plaques in the coronary arteries was usually greater in EHI.

Cases with stenosis of the coronary arteries of more than 50 % of the lumen were less frequent in patients with COPD than in healthy subjects. The differences between the groups with the age-standardized (50–79 years) indices were considerable (17.9 % and 13.9 %) for males; there were no differences between the corresponding groups of females (9.5 % and 8.8 %).

CONCLUSIONS

The data we have presented show that in patients with COPD the development of atherosclerotic changes in various vessels has certain characteristics. An intensification of the atherosclerotic process in the thoracic aorta of patients with COPD is one of the features of the development of atherosclerosis in these patients; the maximal differences between the groups were revealed by an analysis of the frequency and also by comparison of the area of raised lesions.

The degree of atherosclerosis in the abdominal aorta in COPD patients and EHI was practically the same. This was revealed by an analysis of the frequency and the area of fibrous plaques, complicated lesions, and calcification. In contrast to these changes, the area with lipidosis in the abdominal aorta of EHI was usually considerably larger than in COPD patients.

The intensified development of atherosclerotic changes in the thoracic aorta is probably to a great extent due to local factors, since there was not a similar intensification of the process in the abdominal aorta. The local factors could be chronic inflammation in the lungs, pleura, and the para-aortic tissue, leading to disorders of the lymphatic circulation in these areas.

In the coronary arteries atherosclerosis in the presence of COPD was less pronounced than in healthy people; this was noted in all the indices studied. The low frequency of stenosis of the coronary arteries in patients suffering from COPD supports this finding.

The data show that the differences in the extent of atherosclerosis in the aorta versus the coronary arteries in patients with COPD are more marked than in healthy people. The degree of atherosclerosis in the patients with COPD was significantly greater in the thoracic aorta, but less in the coronary arteries, than in EHI. The differences between the two groups of males were considerably greater than the differences between the corresponding groups of females, although the changes were always in the same direction. These features of the development of atherosclerosis in COPD patients should be taken into account when examining atherosclerosis in different groups of people. Elucidation of the facts responsible for the different rates of the development of atherosclerosis in males and females with COPD requires a separate study.

Similarly there is decrease in the area of vessels occupied by fatty streaks in patients with COPD compared to EHI groups. This difference probably results from hypocholesterolemia and hypotension, which are frequently present in these patients (Mutina, 1968; Goryachkina, 1970).

There were no significant differences between the groups in the area of calcification in the coronary arteries. However, COPD patients had a considerably smaller area with fibrous plaques (particularly in males). There is a greater tendency toward calcium deposition in those plaques.

Histological examinations that we conducted (Zhdanov *et al.*, 1973) showed that in some diseases, including COPD, there are reductions in the amount of fats in atherosclerotic plaques. This favors sclerosis and calcium deposition.

Most investigators attribute the inhibitory effect of COPD on the development of atherosclerosis to a number of factors (hypocholesterolemia, hypotension, hypoxia, and emaciation). The differing courses of the atherosclerotic process in vessels studied in those with COPD indicate that the same factors may show different effects on the course of atherosclerosis in different arteries. The effect of hypoxia is most important in the coronary arteries; there it causes an increase in the coronary circulation and dilatation of the coronary vessels. This effect is considered to be one reason for the very slow development of coronary atherosclerosis in patients with COPD (Smolenskii, 1960b; Kolomoiskaya, 1964; Shalevich and Sarankin, 1962).

In patients with COPD the clotting system is often compromised (the coagulation process is decreased and fibrinolytic activity is increased). This may also be a reason for the very slow development of coronary atherosclerosis in patients with this disease (Il'yasov, 1966; Yushina, 1967; Evdokimov, 1968). This hypothesis is supported by our data. Fibrin was very rarely detected on the surface or in the interior of the atherosclerotic plaques in these patients.

At the present time advances in the treatment of COPD have led to a more benign course and extended the lives of patients with this condition. Acute diseases with extensive pulmonary suppuration and marked symptoms that have an inhibitory effect on the development of atherosclerosis (hypocholesterolemia, hypotension, cachexia) are becoming rare. These changes suggest that patients with a combination of COPD and marked degrees of atherosclerosis will be seen more frequently in the future.

8

Atherosclerosis and Chronic Pulmonary Tuberculosis

Interest in the study of the relationship between atherosclerosis and pulmonary tuberculosis has increased appreciably in the last two decades. This can be explained by the increase in the life span of patients with tuberculosis (Braude, 1963, 1966; Il'inskii and Nalimov, 1966; Vail, 1966; Kazykhanov, 1967). Khasanov (1959) presented data showing a nearly threefold increase in the frequency (from 7.0 to 19.1 %) of combinations of pulmonary tuberculosis with atherosclerosis and hypertension in the postwar period as compared to prewar times. According to Vail the advances in treatment of tuberculosis that have prolonged the life of patients are the main cause for the more frequent detection of atherosclerosis in patients of tuberculosis after World War II. According to his data the frequency of the combination of pulmonary tuberculosis with atherosclerosis in 1932–1934 was 11 % versus 28 % now.

The combination of pulmonary tuberculosis with atherosclerosis is usually noted in patients over 40 years of age, which shows the role of age in the rise in frequency of such combinations. The frequency of atherosclerosis in patients with tuberculosis, according to Il'inskii and Nalimov (1966), results not only from the prolongation of life but also from other factors such as diet and the nature of treatment, particularly the administration of vitamin D and prolonged treatment with antibiotics.

The pathological data concerning the characteristics of atherosclerosis in pulmonary tuberculosis are contradictory. Nevertheless, most authors have concluded that atherosclerotic changes are rarely seen in pulmonary tuberculosis and, when present, they are less marked than in other patients. In an analysis of the pathological data from Leningrad Sipovskii and Vlasova (1961) found that the diagnosis of atherosclerosis had been made in only 18 % of the cases of pulmonary tuberculosis (fewer than in COPD, peptic ulcer, malignant tumors, and other diseases). This is probably due to the younger age of the patients with tuberculosis. It has been shown in many studies that the development of atherosclerosis is much slower in patients with pulmonary tuberculosis than in other patients (Rogers, 1957; Grosse, 1960; Weicksel, 1960; Henschen, 1961; Kazykhanov, 1967; Straus *et al.*, 1962; Haber and Marton, 1963; Lashchetko, 1964). Atherosclerotic heart diseases are rare in patients with pulmonary tuberculosis. Straus *et al.* (1962), during prolonged observation of 3,997 patients of pulmonary tuberculosis, noted that atherosclerotic heart diseases could be considered the cause of death in only 0.27%, while in those who did not suffer from pulmonary tuberculosis, they were found three times more frequently (0.8%).

Several authors (Kerner, 1930; Braude, 1963, 1966; Alekseeva, 1966; Restrepo *et al.*, 1968) concluded that there is no inhibitory or suppressing effect of pulmonary tuberculosis on the development of atherosclerotic changes. In their opinion atherosclerosis in these patients develops independently but parallel to pulmonary tuberculosis. However, an analysis of the data provided by these authors does not support this statement. Alekseeva reports that atherosclerosis in different stages was noted in only 22.4% of the cases with tuberculosis. In the remaining 77.6% of the cases with tuberculosis, according to her data, no atherosclerotic changes were present. Alekseeva's data support the presence of a suppressive effect of pulmonary tuberculosis on atherosclerosis. The complete absence of atherosclerosis in such a high percentage of cases gives rise to doubts about the study.

Braude's data are also not convincing. In subjects dying from pulmonary tuberculosis over 40 years of age he observed marked atherosclerosis in 25.1% of the cases. In his opinion this coincides with Anichkov's data (1935). Anichkov noted pronounced atherosclerosis in gross pathological specimens in 25% of the subjects over 40 years of age. Braude therefore maintains that the widely accepted belief in the antagonistic relationships between atherosclerosis and tuberculosis is now untenable and should be considered a thing of the past. To support this conclusion Braude should have compared his data not with Anichkov's, which are 30 years old, but with recent autopsy materials, since not only has the group of patients suffering from tuberculosis changed, but changes have also occurred in the general population. Also it is not clear which vessels were examined by Braude, and it is known that the rates of development of atherosclerosis vary considerably in different vessels. In addition, according to Braude different types and degrees of atherosclerosis were present in only 53.8% of the patients over 40 years of age with pulmonary tuberculosis. In about half of the patients with tuberculosis no atherosclerotic changes were noted in the autopsy reports; this is a highly dubious finding. These facts make the conclusions expressed by Braude of doubtful value.

Anichkov (1935) analyzed autopsy reports from more than 48,000 autopsies in various countries and found data on atherosclerosis in pulmonary tuberculosis in only two reports (from Vienna and Japan). According to Anichkov these reports did not show any significant difference in the degree of atherosclerosis between patients with tuberculosis and other patients.

The morphometric study of atherosclerosis in the aorta and coronary arteries presented by Restrepo *et al.* (1968) did not reveal significant differences in the degree of atherosclerosis between patients with pulmonary tuberculosis and other patients. It is important, however, to note that the authors excluded subjects with atherosclerotic heart diseases, hypertension, or diabetes from the control group.

A number of workers noted intense atherosclerosis in patients with pulmonary tuberculosis (Il'inskii and Nalimov, 1966; Nepryakhin and Akhmetzyanov, 1966). In the opinion of Nepryakhin and Akhmetzyanov there is a relationship between the pathogenesis of chronic pulmonary tuberculosis and atherosclerosis, and this is responsible for the early, rapid development of the accompanying atherosclerosis. The authors noted an intensification of atherosclerotic changes with increasing duration and severity of tuberculosis. In tuberculosis they often found various nonspecific dystrophic changes, mainly in the adventitia of the aorta, lymphoid cell infiltration around the vasa vasorum of the arterial walls, and nonspecific endoperivasculitis of the arterioles.

Kazykhanov (1967) presented contradictory data showing the importance of the duration and severity of tuberculosis in the development of atherosclerosis. During analysis of his own materials Kazykhanov noted that the more extensive and long-standing the pulmonary tuberculosis, the less marked were the atherosclerotic changes in the vessels. According to his data, in those dying from chronic fibrocavernous tuberculosis of the lungs with frequent and prolonged exacerbations atherosclerotic changes were present in 29.7% of the cases, with severe changes in 7.5% of the cases. In other forms of tuberculosis (casevous pneumonia, acute and subacute miliary tuberculosis, fibroid tuberculosis) atherosclerosis of any type was more frequent (46.4%), and severe changes were also more commonly encountered (16.6%).

The above data indicate that in a study of the relationship between tuberculosis and atherosclerosis both the duration and the nature (severity) of tuberculosis have some significance. Modern therapy for tuberculosis is responsible for the favorable course of the disease and the increase in the average life span of tuberculosis patients. At present many patients with pulmonary tuberculosis do not die directly from a progressive tubercular process but from its complications (for example, cardiopulmonary failure) or from other diseases.

Many authors attribute the retarded development of atherosclerosis in patients with pulmonary tuberculosis to a series of complex factors: disorders of lipid and protein metabolism, hypotension, hypoxia, and cachexia.

Our attention is drawn to the frequent presence of changes in lipid metabolism (Rosenthal, 1934; Medvedeva, 1955; Straus *et al.*, 1962; Kazykhanov,

1967). Hypocholesterolemia, a rise in the level of β-lipoproteins, and a fall in the level of α-lipoproteins are often observed in patients with pulmonary tuberculosis.

Hypotension is a characteristic for patients with pulmonary tuberculosis (Weicksel, 1960; Haber and Marton, 1963; Gerasimchuk, 1966), which is often observed in patients with severe forms of the disease (Benians, 1956; Kazykhanov, 1967). It has frequently been noted (Shmelev, 1957; Kulachkovskii, 1967) that hypotension in these patients is at least partly due to adrenal insufficiency.

Histological and histochemical studies have demonstrated that the atherosclerotic changes in pulmonary tuberculosis are nonspecific (Kremlev, 1951; Akhmetzyanov, 1967). There are, however, quantitative differences in the degree of different types of change: fatty streaks, fibrous plaques, complicated lesions, and calcification.

We studied the degree of atherosclerosis in the aorta and coronary arteries in 318 patients who died from chronic pulmonary tuberculosis (Table 37). The pathological diagnosis in most cases was bilateral fibrocavernous tuberculosis of the lungs. Cases with primary tuberculous lesions in other organs (for example, in the kidneys, sex organs, or bones) or cases with minor tuberculous changes in the lungs in combination with other diseases were not included in the study.

Table 37. Age and Sex Distribution of Chronic Pulmonary Tuberculosis Cases

Age in years	20–29	30–39	40–49	50–59	60–69	Total
Males	22	44	44	48	31	189
Females	19	36	18	24	22	129

Changes with age in atherosclerosis in the aorta and coronary arteries in patients with chronic pulmonary tuberculosis were identical to those observed in other groups.

The frequency of lesions, the total area with atherosclerotic changes, and the area with raised lesions increased with age. In most cases in the third or fourth decade of life in the aorta and coronary arteries only fatty streaks were present; beginning with the fifth decade of life there were fatty streaks in combination with fibrous plaques. In patients with chronic pulmonary tuberculosis uniform atherosclerosis in the different parts of the aorta was noted, since the degree of atherosclerosis in the thoracic aorta, particularly in the fifth and sixth decades of life, was similar to that in the abdominal aorta. In males with chronic pulmonary tuberculosis, atherosclerotic changes in the coronary arteries usually occupied a considerably larger area than in females;

Table 38. Mean Area of Atherosclerotic Changes in Patients with Chronic Pulmonary Tuberculosis

Age in years	Total cases	Statistical values	Abdominal aorta					Left anterior descending coronary artery				
			TA	F	FbPl	Co	Ca	TA	F	FbPl	Co	Ca
Males												
20–29	22	M	16.5	13.2	3.0	0.1	0.1	7.6	2.6	4.9	0.0	0.05
		SE	3.3	3.3	1.4	0.1	0.1	1.5	0.9	1.5	0.0	0.04
30–39	44	M	20.9	13.7	7.0	0.04	0.1	11.7	2.2	8.9	0.02	0.6
		SE	2.0	2.0	1.7	0.03	0.1	1.6	0.4	1.4	0.03	0.2
40–49	44	M	30.4	9.2	19.7	0.6	0.9	19.2	2.7	15.7	0.02	0.7
		SE	3.1	2.3	2.6	0.3	0.5	2.2	0.6	2.1	0.03	0.6
50–59	48	M	42.6	6.8	31.7	1.4	2.7	34.4	2.0	27.7	0.1	4.6
		SE	2.9	1.2	2.4	0.3	0.9	3.2	0.3	2.6	0.05	1.3
60–69	31	M	49.9	5.9	39.3	2.5	2.2	31.6	2.8	24.9	0.03	3.8
		SE	3.6	2.0	3.2	1.0	1.3	4.3	0.5	4.0	0.04	2.8
Females												
20–29	19	M	18.0	15.9	2.1	0.0	0.0	4.9	2.3	2.6	0.0	0.0
		SE	2.4	2.9	1.1	0.0	0.0	1.3	0.6	1.2	0.0	0.0
30–39	36	M	25.0	16.2	8.7	0.05	0.02	7.3	1.8	5.5	0.0	0.0
		SE	1.9	2.2	3.4	0.1	0.03	1.5	0.3	1.4	0.0	0.0
40–49	18	M	31.5	13.0	17.9	0.3	0.3	14.0	2.7	11.2	0.0	0.1
		SE	6.3	3.3	5.9	0.3	0.2	4.9	0.8	4.9	0.0	0.1
50–59	24	M	42.6	10.7	28.5	1.7	1.7	13.9	3.1	10.1	0.0	0.3
		SE	3.7	2.9	3.8	1.5	0.7	2.7	0.4	3.1	0.0	0.1
60–69	22	M	38.4	4.8	29.2	0.5	3.8	24.7	1.9	14.5	0.0	8.3
		SE	5.2	1.1	0.3	0.2	0.3	4.8	0.2	3.9	0.0	3.1

* TA, total area with atherosclerotic change; F, fatty streaks; FbPl, fibrous plaques; Co, complicated lesions; Ca, calcification; M, mean; SE, standard error. Area given as a percentage of intimal surface of vessels.

the maximal differences were noted in the total area of atherosclerotic changes and the area with raised lesions. In the aorta the differences between males and females in the degree of atherosclerosis were insignificant, but a tendency to a greater area with raised lesions was observed in males (Table 38).

Stenosis of the coronary arteries by 50% or more in males with chronic pulmonary tuberculosis was noted in the sixth and seventh decades of life (11.3% and 22.6% of the cases, respectively), and in female patients only in the seventh decade of life (13.3% of the cases).

PREVALENCE OF ATHEROSCLEROTIC CHANGES IN TUBERCULOSIS PATIENTS AND IN EHI

In all groups the aorta had fatty streaks in combination with fibrous plaques by the third decade of life. In the subsequent decade in all groups the number of cases with fatty streaks only in the aorta decreased and the number of cases with fibrous plaques, complicated lesions, and/or calcification rapidly increased.

In the thoracic aorta of essentially healthy males fatty streaks were noted more frequently (the differences were statistically significant in the fifth, sixth, and seventh decades of life and in the age-standardized indices) than in patients with pulmonary tuberculosis. The differences between the groups in the prevalence of fibrous plaques, complicated lesions, and/or calcification were not statistically significant. Therefore, one can only say that a marked tendency exists. The differences between the corresponding groups of females in the prevalence of the various types of atherosclerotic changes in thoracic aorta were not significant (Table 39).

In the abdominal aorta of patients with pulmonary tuberculosis complicated lesions and/or calcification were frequently noted, while in healthy people fatty streaks in combination with fibrous plaques were more common. The differences between the corresponding groups of males were often statistically significant both for individual decades of life and in the age-standardized index. The differences between the corresponding groups of females were statistically significant only for individual decades of life.

In both groups the coronary arteries had no grossly visible atherosclerotic changes. These were noted more frequently in males with pulmonary tuberculosis (Table 39). The differences in the frequency of various types of atherosclerotic changes in the coronary arteries were usually small. Nevertheless, on the basis of age-standardized indices, males with pulmonary tuberculosis demonstrated more complicated lesions and/or calcification in the coronary arteries. In healthy individuals lipidosis alone or lipidosis in combination with fibrous plaques were more frequent. In females the differences between the groups were smaller; only in the right coronary artery were complicated lesions and/or calcification seen significantly more frequently in essentially healthy females (Table 39).

Table 39. Age-standardized (20–69 years) Indices of Frequency of Atherosclerotic Changes in EHI (1) and Patients with Chronic Pulmonary Tuberculosis (2)

Types of changes	Groups	ThA	AA	RCA	LCCA	LADCA
Males						
No change	1	—	—	11.2	15.9	3.9
	2	—	—	18.5*	21.8*	8.9*
Lipidosis only	1	44.2	29.6	28.7	25.9	16.8
	2	36.7*	24.4	20.3*	22.0	14.0
Lipidosis and fibrous plaques	1	41.1	41.3	47.0	49.6	62.1
	2	45.0	34.8*	46.3	47.4	55.4*
Complicated lesions and calcification	1	14.2	29.0	13.1	8.6	17.2
	2	17.4	38.9*	14.3	8.6	21.6
Females						
No change	1	—	—	18.1	18.6	6.6
	2	—	—	22.7	24.0	7.2
Lipidosis only	1	46.4	35.0	35.2	40.3	28.5
	2	47.8	34.7	36.8	40.4	29.7
Lipidosis and fibrous plaques	1	41.8	43.5	35.5	36.3	52.7
	2	38.4	37.9	36.6	30.8	53.5
Complicated lesions and calcification	1	11.5	21.5	9.9	4.8	12.1
	2	13.8	27.4	3.9*	4.8	9.5

ThA, thoracic aorta; AA, abdominal aorta; RCA, right coronary artery; LCCA, left circumflex coronary artery; LADCA, left anterior descending coronary artery.

* Differences statistically significant ($p \leqslant 0.05$). Frequency given as percentage of change in vessels.

COMPARISON OF ATHEROSCLEROTIC AREAS IN EHI AND PATIENTS WITH PULMONARY TUBERCULOSIS

In both parts of the aorta the total area with atherosclerotic changes, particularly the area with raised lesions, was often larger in the group of patients with chronic pulmonary tuberculosis (Fig. 29, Table 40). However, in the individual decades of life the differences between the groups were rarely statistically significant. The age-standardized index for the area with raised lesions in the aorta revealed statistically significant differences between the corresponding groups of females.

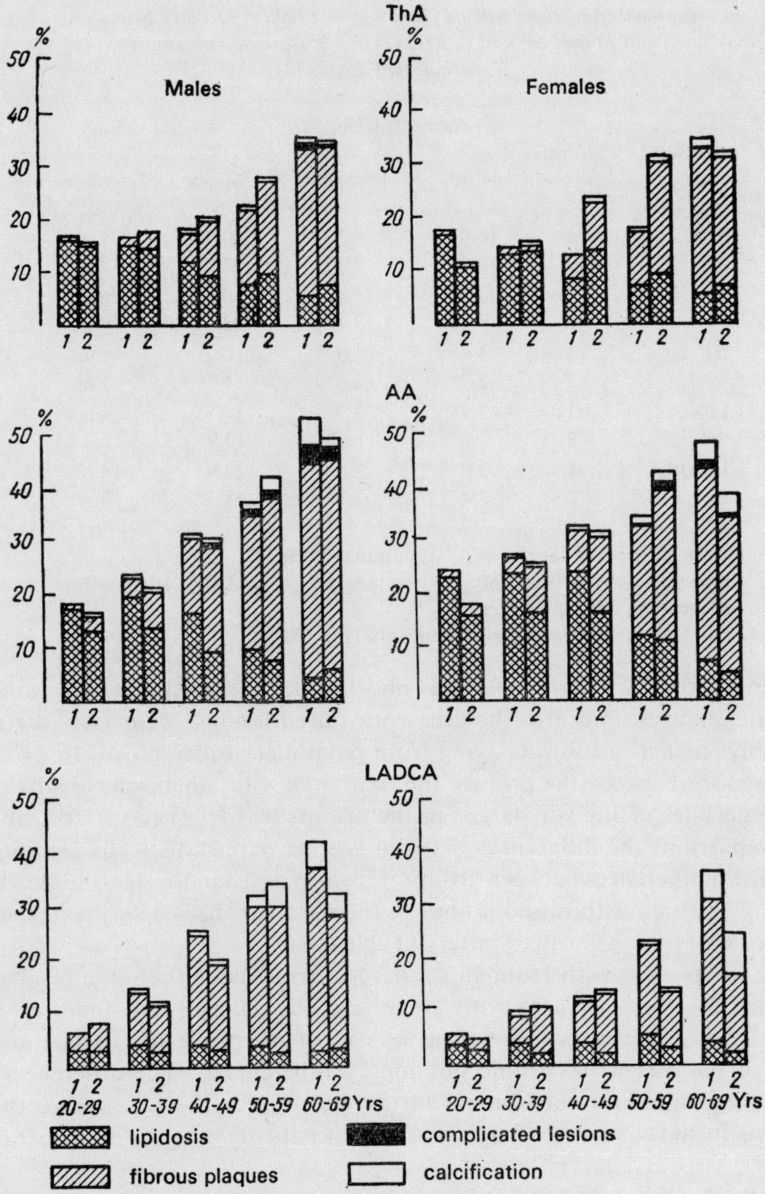

Figure 29. Characteristics of atherosclerosis in healthy subjects (*1*) and in patients with pulmonary tuberculosis (*2*). Ordinate shows changed area as a percentage of the intimal surface of the vessels. ThA, thoracic aorta; AA, abdominal aorta; LADCA, left anterior descending coronary artery.

Table 40. Age-standardized (20–69 years) Indices of Fatty Streaks and Raised Lesions in EHI (1) and in Chronic Pulmonary Tuberculosis Patients (2)

Vessels	Groups	Fatty streaks		Raised lesions	
		Males	Females	Males	Females
ThA	1	10.9	9.7	10.5	8.9
	2	10.9	9.9*	12.2	12.0*
AA	1	12.8	17.2	19.6	16.0
	2	9.8*	12.1*	22.3	19.0*
RCA	1	3.8	4.0	16.9	9.9
	2	2.9*	2.5*	14.2*	5.6*
LCCA	1	3.2	3.7	14.5	9.0
	2	2.2*	1.6*	13.9	6.4
LADCA	1	3.0	3.6	22.9	13.6
	2	2.4	2.3*	18.5*	10.5*

ThA, thoracic aorta; AA, abdominal aorta; RCA, right coronary artery; LCCA, left circumflex coronary artery; LADCA, left anterior descending coronary artery.

* Differences statistically significant ($p \leqslant 0.05$).

In the coronary arteries of males and females the total area with atherosclerotic changes, and also the area with raised lesions, were as a rule considerably smaller in subjects dying from pulmonary tuberculosis. In 24 of 34 comparisons between the groups, the total area with atherosclerosis by individual decades of life was larger in the groups of EHI ($p_{kz} < 0.01$), and in 11 comparisons the differences between groups were statistically significant. Significant differences between groups were also noted in the age-standardized index of the area with raised lesions in the right coronary artery and the left anterior descending coronary artery (Table 40).

When expressed with Holman's atherosclerotic index the same results are obtained for the total area with atherosclerotic changes and the area with raised lesions. The index shows great severity of atherosclerosis in the thoracic aorta of patients with chronic pulmonary tuberculosis. The differences between the groups in the abdominal aorta were not great. The degree of atherosclerosis in the coronary arteries was less in patients with pulmonary tuberculosis.

Analysis of the data for individual types of atherosclerotic change similarly reveals characteristic differences between the groups. Regarding the area with fatty streaks in the thoracic aorta, the differences between the groups were not in the same direction in various decades. The changes were statistically significant only in some decades of life. In all the remaining vessels studied (abdominal aorta and coronary arteries) the area with fatty streaks was usually considerably smaller in subjects with tuberculosis; this was noted during comparison of groups by the decade of life and in the age-standardized index (Fig. 29, Table 40). In the abdominal aorta and coronary arteries, 40 comparisons were made between the groups by decades of life. In 37 comparisons the area with lipidosis was larger in a group of EHI, and in only three individuals with chronic pulmonary tuberculosis was it larger ($p_{Kz} < 0.01$).

Fibrous plaques as a rule occupied a larger area of both parts of the aorta in patients with pulmonary tuberculosis than in the healthy individuals (this occurred in 16 of 20 comparisons by decades of life; $p_{Kz} = 0.01$). The age-standardized (20–69 years) indices for the area with fibrous plaques also showed very high values for patients with pulmonary tuberculosis. In the coronary arteries the area with fibrous plaques was considerably smaller in patients with pulmonary tuberculosis. This difference was noted both during comparison of groups by individual decades of life and in the age-standardized index.

There were no significant differences between groups in the area of the coronary arteries with calcification, although the area with fibrous plaques was usually smaller in patients with pulmonary tuberculosis. From these data it can be concluded that there is a greater tendency for deposition of calcium in fibrous plaques in the patients with tuberculosis.

CONCLUSIONS

This study of atherosclerotic changes in the aorta and coronary arteries in chronic pulmonary tuberculosis has revealed certain features of the development of atherosclerosis in various vessels. In the thoracic aorta atherosclerosis was usually more marked in those with pulmonary tuberculosis than in the healthy. This was indicated by the greater frequency and the larger area with atherosclerotic changes (total area of atherosclerotic changes, area with fibrous plaques, total area with raised lesions) and by the higher atherosclerotic index for the group with tuberculosis.

Some intensification of atherosclerotic changes in the thoracic aorta is possibly due to the local effect of pulmonary changes on the aorta. This was mentioned in the discussion of atherosclerosis in the aorta in chronic non-specific inflammatory diseases of the lungs.

In patients with chronic pulmonary tuberculosis there was also a tendency to more marked atherosclerosis in the abdominal aorta than in EHI. The data showing the prevalence and area with raised lesions support this statement. In some comparisons the total area of atherosclerotic changes in the abdominal aorta was somewhat smaller in those with pulmonary tuberculosis than in EHI. However, this was due to the less extensive fatty streaks and plaques in these patients. The data presented here showing the characteristics of the development of atherosclerosis in the aorta in patients with chronic pulmonary tuberculosis support Akhmetzyanov's data (1967) indicating intensification of the atherosclerotic process in the aorta of such patients.

The degree of atherosclerosis in the coronary arteries was usually considerably less in the group of patients with tuberculosis than in healthy people. This has been noted by others (Rogers, 1957; Weicksel, 1960; Lashchetko, 1964; Kazykhanov, 1967; Straus *et al.*, 1962).

These data show various tendencies of the development of atherosclerosis in the aorta and coronary arteries in patients with pulmonary tuberculosis. They suggest that the so-called inhibitory factors (hypocholesterolemia, hypotension, hypoxia, and cachexia) in fact take part in the development of atherosclerosis in the coronary arteries. In those suffering from chronic pulmonary tuberculosis the area of the aorta with fatty streaks is smaller than in a control group of healthy people; the areas of other types of atherosclerotic changes were either the same in both groups or larger in patients with chronic pulmonary tuberculosis. The decrease in the area of lipidosis in the vessels studied in all probability is due to the hypocholesterolemia often found in patients with chronic pulmonary tuberculosis (Naugol'nova, 1964; Kazykhanov, 1967; Straus *et al.*, 1962). This is also in agreement with the histochemical data of Kremnev (1951) and the biochemical studies by Eilerson and Faber (1960), who showed a decrease in the deposition of cholesterol in the aorta in pulmonary tuberculosis. Kremnev showed the regression of atherosclerotic changes in the aorta in emaciating diseases, mostly due to resorption of fatty streaks.

The area with calcification in the vessels studied in comparable groups was basically the same or somewhat larger in patients with pulmonary tuberculosis. In particular, this was found in the coronary arteries. The total area with atherosclerosis and the area with fibrous plaques in the coronary arteries were often considerably smaller in patients with pulmonary tuberculosis, but calcification was relatively more marked in these patients than in EHI. These data indicate that calcification of the vessels is not solely dependent on the degree of atherosclerosis. Eilerson and Faber (1960) noted a decrease in the accumulation of lipids in the aorta in pulmonary tuberculosis. They emphasized that accumulation of calcium in this situation continues throughout the period of emaciation. Hypoxia is probably one of the factors favoring calcification. This view is to some extent supported by the experimental findings of Saefer *et al.* (1961).

Our data regarding the characteristics of the development of atherosclerosis in patients with chronic pulmonary tuberculosis are quite similar to the data regarding the development of the atherosclerotic process in patients with chronic, nonspecific inflammatory diseases of the lungs (see chapter 7). To a great extent this stems from the similar changes in lipid metabolism in these groups of patients from the tendency to hypotension, and from the emaciation and hypoxia that are often noted in both groups of patients. The cause of death in these patients is also more or less the same (pulmonary or cardio-pulmonary failure) and generally results from fibrotic changes in the lungs.

In conclusion, the advances in the treatment of pulmonary tuberculosis in the last two or three decades have led to a considerable prolongation of the average span of life of patients with tuberculosis. This is one of the main reasons for the increased prevalence of cases showing a combination of atherosclerosis and chronic pulmonary tuberculosis.

9

Atherosclerosis and Thyrotoxicosis

The disorders of lipid, carbohydrate, and protein metabolism have an important effect on the pathogenesis of atherosclerosis. Diseases of the endocrine glands cause important metabolic changes. A study of the interrelationship between the degree of atherosclerosis and thyroid function shows a considerable effect of thyroid hormones on the development of atherosclerosis. Adequate data have now accumulated to show that hypothyroidism is usually associated with accelerated atherosclerosis, and hyperthyroidism is characterized by a delay in the development of atherosclerosis (Fridlyand, 1927; Tatarskii and Tsinzerling, 1950; Sharlai, 1958; Myasnikov, 1960, 1965; Avtsyn *et al.*, 1961; Boyd, 1961; Myasnikov and Pyatenko, 1962; Myant, 1964; Roguski *et al.*, 1964; Myasnikov *et al.*, 1967; Myasnikov, 1969). However, there are very few studies based on the morphological characteristics of goiter in a large post-mortem series (Welsch *et al.*, 1961; Yagudaev, 1968; Yusupov, 1971; Aleksandrov, 1973).

The characteristics of the development of different types of atherosclerotic changes with various functional disorders of the thyroid gland have yet to be adequately studied. In some studies the prevalence of atherosclerotic changes has been presented without comparison with a control group.

Goldschmidt (1934) analyzed autopsy materials in 115 subjects between 40 and 70 years old who died with Basedow's disease. He noted that in these subjects atherosclerosis was rarer and less pronounced than in those dying from other diseases. Only 40.8% of the subjects with Basedow's disease showed atherosclerotic changes (often these were mild); in subjects dying from other diseases atherosclerotic changes had been noticed in 99% of the autopsy reports.

Other workers (Myasnikov and Pyatenko, 1962; Gurova and Abramova, 1965; Kushelevskii and Gurova, 1966) observed an extensive, severe atherosclerosis in some patients with thyrotoxicosis. It is important to note that in these cases the duration of thyrotoxicosis was not long. It is possible that these patients had severe atherosclerosis prior to the development of thyrotoxicosis. When studying atherosclerosis in patients with thyrotoxicosis it is important to consider not only the age of the patient but also the duration of thyrotoxicosis. There is usually an inverse relationship between the degree of atherosclerosis and the duration of thyrotoxicosis (Gurova and Abramova, 1965).

A number of investigators emphasize the great rarity of myocardial infarction in patients with thyrotoxicosis, which is undoubtedly explained by the very low degree of atherosclerotic changes in the coronary arteries (Burstein *et al.*, 1960; Parashchak and Shvedenko, 1963; Kushelevskii and Gurova, 1966). Gritting and Salvesen (1957) noted coronary disease (without myocardial infarction) in only one of 521 patients with thyrotoxicosis. In 15 patients mild or moderate atherosclerotic changes were present. Often the coronary arteries were completely free of disease. The authors concluded that in long-standing thyrotoxicosis the coronary arteries have little atherosclerosis, even in elderly people.

Yagudaev (1968) conducted interesting studies of the relationship between atherosclerosis in the aorta and the histological and functional characteristics of the thyroid gland in the population of an endemic area. The rates of development of atherosclerosis were high in subjects with diffuse colloidal and sclerotic types of goiter, and low in nodular goiters, where the follicles were small but filled with colloid. In the former, the histological picture indicated minimal activity of the thyroid gland; in the latter, very high activity of the thyroid gland nodules in comparison with the surrounding glandular tissue. These data demonstrate that in studying the effect of endemic goiter on the development of atherosclerosis it is necessary to consider the morphological appearance and functional activity of the thyroid. This should be kept in mind when considering the findings of Welsch *et al.* (1961), who found no correlation between colloidal goiter and atherosclerosis in the aorta and coronary arteries. These authors did not consider the functional activity of the thyroid gland in a group of patients with colloidal goiter. The study probably included cases with both increased and decreased thyroid activity.

Most investigators attribute the effect of thyroid hormones on the development of atherosclerosis to their action on lipid metabolism (Rosenman *et al.*, 1952; Il'inskii, 1960; Myasnikov, 1960, 1965; Myant, 1964; Leites, 1967; Tagi-Zade, 1967; Myasnikov, 1969). In thyrotoxicosis the most important and most commonly noted disorder of lipid metabolism is a fall in serum cholesterol and its fractions; similarly there is a tendency for the level of total lipids and phospholipids to fall. Only in isolated cases of thyrotoxicosis are there disorders of the lipid metabolism that closely resemble those of patients with atherosclerosis (Myasnikov and Pyatenko, 1962). It should be noted that these cases are very rare, and in some of them thyrotoxicosis has developed in the presence of atherosclerosis.

Many authors have recently suggested that the hypocholesterolemic effect of the thyroid hormones is due to their action on the cholesterol metabolism of the liver. This has been demonstrated under experimental conditions (Myasnikov and Klemashev, 1965, 1969; Rosenman *et al.*, 1952; Fletcher and Myant, 1962; Myasnikov *et al.*, 1967; Myasnikov, 1969). Administration of thyroxin to animals with atherosclerosis produced an accumulation of cholesterol in the liver, a fall in cholesterol in the blood and aorta, and a rise in the excretion of cholesterol in the bile. Damage to the liver with carbon tetrachloride completely neutralizes the effect of thyroxin on the cholesterol levels in the blood, liver, and aorta. In partial and completely hepatectomized animals the thyroid hormones also have no action on the blood cholesterol level (Page, cited by Myasnikov, 1965).

The metabolism effects of thyroid hormones operate not only through the liver but also through other organs. Myasnikov *et al.* (1967) have shown that the passage of cholesterol from the blood to the liver is mediated by the reticulo-endothelial cells of the liver. Blockage of these cells with India ink and other substances partially neutralizes the effect of thyroid hormones on the cholesterol metabolism. Thyroxin also causes changes in the activity of lipolytic enzymes (Leites, 1967; Fuks and Leites, 1967), the metabolism of mucopolysaccharide in the vessel wall (Fischer, 1964; Uotila *et al.*, 1961), and the action of sex hormones (Gimbashidze, 1967).

The condition of the thyroid gland in patients with atherosclerosis has also been studied. Ganelina and Komarova (1963) have shown a tendency for the function of the thyroid gland to fall as determined both by basal metabolic studies and by the radioactive iodine method. A decrease in the activity of the thyroid gland is observed in approximately half of the patients; these are mainly patients with severe atherosclerosis. The decrease in function is probably related to atherosclerotic changes in the thyroid gland. In this respect we may cite the studies of Chernokany (1967) who studied histochemical changes in the thyroid gland in the early stages of atherosclerosis. At this stage he found an increased synthesis of thyroid hormone and increased excretion of the secretory products from the follicles. In the cases with pronounced and widespread atherosclerosis the secretory activity of the thyroid gland was suppressed.

The experimental data concerning the changes in the thyroid gland in atherosclerosis are contradictory. Kipshidze (1959) and Vadachkoriya (1964) observed an immediate fall in the activity of the thyroid gland during the experimental production of atherosclerosis. Maksudov (1960) noted this fall only in the late stages of the development of atherosclerosis; Danilova *et al.* (1967) observed only stimulation of the function of the thyroid gland. The comparative data for the changes in the thyroid gland produced by feeding cholesterol to hamsters, rats, rabbits, and guinea pigs are of interest (Bernick *et al.*, 1962). These changes were diverse in nature and correlated well with the degree of experimental atherosclerosis. In hamsters and rats there was hyperplasia of the thyroid and a low degree of atherosclerosis; in rabbits and guinea pigs there was hypoplasia of the thyroid and pronounced atherosclerotic changes. The authors think that the resistance of some animals to atherosclerosis depends to a certain extent on the nature of the reaction of their thyroid gland to cholesterol.

In recent years various disorders in the coagulation and anticoagulation systems of the blood, which are frequently noted in diseases of the thyroid gland, have gained attention in the study of atherosclerosis (Pavloskii and Korvatskii, 1963; Tagi-Zade, 1967). These studies have demonstrated that in thyrotoxicosis there is a prolongation of the clotting time and a rise in the fibrinolytic activity of the blood, i.e., phenomena opposite to those noted in atherosclerosis. In thyrotoxicosis there is prolongation of the clotting time, decreased plasma tolerance to heparin, prolongation of the recalcification time, a drop in the level of fibrinogen, and a rise in the level of free heparin and fibrinolytic activity. Severe forms of thyrotoxicosis are associated with more severe changes in the clotting system. These changes in the clotting system in thyrotoxicosis are probably an important cause of the inhibition of atherosclerosis in thyrotoxicosis.

We studied the degree of atherosclerosis in 60 females and in 3 males with thyrotoxicosis; 3 cases were in the third decade of life, 3 in the fourth, 9 in the fifth, 23 (21 females and 2 males) in the sixth, 22 (21 females and 1 male) in the seventh, and 3 cases in the eighth decade of life. Mean values were calculated only for females in the fifth, sixth, and seventh decades of life. Comparisons were conducted in most cases with a group of EHI. The atherosclerotic changes were always much more pronounced in those dying from the various complications of atherosclerosis than in EHI and in those with thyrotoxicosis.

PREVALENCE OF ATHEROSCLEROTIC CHANGES IN THYROTOXICOSIS PATIENTS AND EHI

In the third decade of life in the patients with thyrotoxicosis (3 cases) only fatty streaks were found in the aorta; fibrous plaques in EHI were sometimes present in the thoracic (13%) and in the abdominal aorta (18.4%).

In five of the nine coronary arteries studied in subjects dying from thyrotoxicosis there were no atherosclerotic changes. In the remaining arteries there were only fatty streaks or fatty streaks in combination with fibrous plaques. In EH females coronary arteries without changes were noted in 31.4%, and with fibrous plaques in 17.9% of the cases.

Only one of the three patients with thyrotoxicosis showed fibrous plaques in the abdominal aorta in the fourth decade of life. In healthy subjects fibrous plaques were frequently present in the abdominal aorta (33.9% of the cases) and also in the thoracic aorta (19.5% of the cases). In two of three cases with thyrotoxicosis there were fatty streaks and fibrous plaques in the coronary arteries. In one case no changes were found in the coronary arteries; in healthy people fibrous plaques were present in the coronary arteries in 60% of the cases.

In the fifth, sixth, and seventh decades of life the prevalence of vessels with fatty streaks and fibrous plaques was greater in patients with thyrotoxicosis. Vessels with complicated lesions and/or calcification were more prevalent in the group of EHI.

The differences between the groups in the prevalence of these changes were more marked for the aorta than for the coronary arteries; in the left anterior descending coronary artery complicated lesions and/or calcification were even noted more frequently in patients with thyrotoxicosis (Table 41).

Table 41. Prevalence of Vascular Changes in EHI (1) and in Females with Thyrotoxicosis (2)

Vessels	Groups	Vessels without changes with lipidosis and fibrous plaques			Vessels with calcification and/ or complicated lesions		
		40–49	50–59	60–69	40–49	50–59	60–69
Abdominal aorta	1	88.3	65.6	41.5	11.7	34.4	58.5
	2	100.0*	85.6*	57.3*	—	14.4*	42.7
Left coronary artery	1	96.0	79.1	64.2	4.0	20.9	35.8
	2	88.9	76.2	60.0	11.1	23.8	40.8

* Differences statistically significant ($p \leqslant 0.05$). Figures given are percentages of cases with changes.

Table 42. Prevalence of Calcification in EHI (1) and Females with Thyrotoxicosis (2)

Vessels	Groups	50–59 yrs	60–69 yrs
Thoracic aorta	1	7.3	28.1
	2	4.8	23.8
Abdominal aorta	1	29.2	42.4
	2	9.6*	42.7
Right coronary artery	1	15.0	18.2
	2	4.8*	15.0
Left coronary artery	1	17.6	34.4
	2	9.5	10.0*

* Differences statistically significant ($p \leqslant 0.05$). Figures given are percentages of cases with changes.

Calcification was more frequent in the vessels of EH females than in those with thyrotoxicosis (Table 42), but these differences were usually not statistically significant.

The data indicate that patients with thyrotoxicosis more frequently have mild degrees of atherosclerosis (vessels with only lipidosis and fibrous plaques); essentially healthy individuals more frequently demonstrated advanced stages of atherosclerosis (vessels with complicated lesions and/or calcification).

COMPARISON OF ATHEROSCLEROTIC AREAS IN EHI AND IN THYROTOXICOSIS PATIENTS

The total area of atherosclerotic changes in the thoracic aorta in both the groups in the fifth, sixth, and seventh decades of life did not differ, although the ratios of individual types of changes were somewhat different in these groups. In the abdominal aorta and coronary arteries the total area of changes in patients with thyrotoxicosis was considerably smaller than in EHI (Fig. 30), and these differences were statistically significant in the sixth and seventh decades of life.

Holman's atherosclerosis index, which is calculated on the basis of all types of change, was lower for the abdominal aorta and coronary arteries in patients with thyrotoxicosis; the index for the thoracic aorta was almost the same in both groups. Atherosclerotic changes occupied a considerably larger area and the index was highest (Fig. 31) in subjects dying from various complications of atherosclerosis.

The area of the aorta and coronary arteries with lipidosis in those with thyrotoxicosis was usually considerably less than in EHI (Fig. 30). The statistically significant differences between the groups in respect to the area with lipidosis were found in the thoracic aorta in the sixth and seventh decades of life; in the abdominal aorta in the fifth, sixth, and seventh decades of life; in the left anterior descending coronary artery in the sixth; and in the left circumflex coronary artery in the fifth and sixth decades of life.

The area occupied by fibrous plaques in the thoracic aorta in those with thyrotoxicosis was the same or even higher than in EHI. In all the remaining vessels fibrous plaques in patients with thyrotoxicosis were considerably less extensive than in a control group of healthy people. The difference between the groups in respect to the area occupied by fibrous plaques in the aorta was not statistically significant; for the coronary arteries, these differences were statistically significant in most cases.

Complicated lesions did not occupy a large area in either group; these changes were usually extensive in the abdominal aorta and coronary arteries in EHI, but in the thoracic aorta there were no differences between the

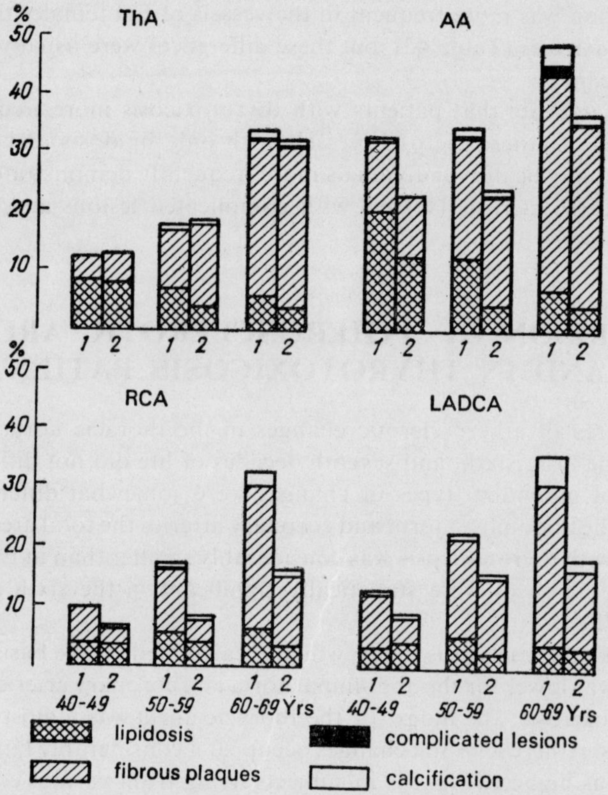

Figure 30. Characteristics of atherosclerosis in vessels in healthy individuals (*1*) and in female patients with thyrotoxicosis (*2*). Ordinate shows changed area as percentage of intimal surface of vessels. ThA, thoracic aorta; AA, abdominal aorta; RCA, right coronary artery; LADCA, left anterior descending coronary artery.

groups. In patients with thyrotoxicosis complicated lesions were noted only after the sixth, and in EH females after the fifth, decade of life. In the coronary arteries the mean area with complicated lesions in both the groups in the sixth and seventh decades of life did not exceed 0.3 % of the intimal surface. Complicated changes were maximal in the abdominal aorta; in EH females of 50 to 59 years of age they constituted $0.4 \pm 0.1\%$ of the area; in those 60 to 69 years of age, $1.3 \pm 0.5\%$. In patients with thyrotoxicosis they occupied $0.1 \pm 0.06\%$ and $0.1 \pm 0.06\%$ of the intimal surface, respectively ($p < 0.05$).

The area with calcification was smaller in patients with thyrotoxicosis than in EHI. The differences between the groups were the smallest in the fifth and

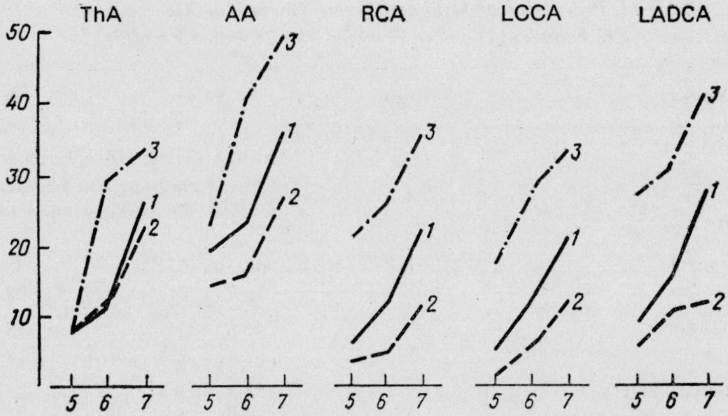

Figure 31. The atherosclerotic index for vessels in healthy females (*1*), patients with thyrotoxicosis (*2*), and those dying from atherosclerosis (*3*). ThA, thoracic aorta; AA, abdominal aorta; RCA, right coronary artery; LCCA, left circumflex coronary artery; LADCA, left anterior descending coronary artery.

the largest in the seventh decade of life (Fig. 30). In all the vessels studied the differences between the groups in the area of calcification were statistically significant.

In those with thyrotoxicosis the total area with raised lesions in the abdominal aorta and coronary arteries was smaller than in EHI; these differences increased with age and were greatest in the seventh decade of life. In the thoracic aorta the above changes were of more or less the same extent in both groups.

The groups were also compared with regard to the stages of atherosclerosis: mild atherosclerosis, raised lesions occupying not more than 15% of the intimal surface; moderate, 15% to 50%; severe, raised lesions occupy more than 50% of the intimal surface of the vessels. The data support those presented above, in that they show a very slow development of atherosclerosis in patients with thyrotoxicosis. It appears that in these patients vessels with a mild degree of atherosclerosis are observed more frequently, and vessels with a severe degree of atherosclerosis are rarely seen (Table 43).

There was not a single case of thyrotoxicosis in which atherosclerotic changes occupied 75% or more of the intimal surface of the vessels. In EHI 75% or greater involvement with atherosclerosis in the abdominal aorta was noted in 26.3%, and in the left anterior descending coronary artery in 22% of cases. Stenosis of the coronary arteries exceeding 50% of the lumen was present in only one of 21 cases with thyrotoxicosis in the age group 50 to 59 years (4.7%) and in one of 21 cases in the group 60 to 69 years of age (4.7%). In healthy females 50 to 59 years of age stenosis was as rare as in patients with

Table 43. Prevalence of Mild and Severe Degrees of Atherosclerosis in EH Females (1) and in Females with Thyrotoxicosis (2)

Vessels	Groups	50–59 yrs	60–69 yrs
		Mild atherosclerosis (area with fibrous plaques, complicated lesions and calcification less than 15%)	
Thoracic aorta	1	66.3 (237)†	38.0 (150)
	2	66.7 (21)	28.5 (21)
Abdominal aorta	1	46.9 (234)	18.7 (150)
	2	52.4 (21)	18.9 (21)
Right coronary artery	1	53.8 (236)	25.3 (142)
	2	100.0* (21)	80.0* (21)
Left circumflex coronary artery	1	59.0 (227)	40.5 (136)
	2	80.9* (21)	71.4* (21)
Left anterior descending coronary artery	1	34.5 (229)	17.6 (142)
	2	71.4* (21)	60.0* (21)
		Severe atherosclerosis (area with fibrous plaques, complicated lesions and calcification greater than 50%)	
Thoracic aorta	1	8.0 (237)	21.3 (150)
	2	4.7 (21)	14.3 (21)
Abdominal aorta	1	22.7 (234)	48.0 (150)
	2	9.5* (21)	19.1* (21)
Right coronary artery	1	18.1 (236)	33.8 (142)
	2	0.0 (21)	10.0* (20)
Left circumflex coronary artery	1	12.8 (227)	29.4 (136)
	2	0.0 (21)	4.8* (21)
Left anterior descending coronary artery	1	16.0 (229)	30.3 (142)
	2	0.0 (21)	5.0* (21)

* Differences statistically significant ($p \leq 0.05$).

† Figures in brackets are number of observations. Prevalence given as a percentage of observations.

thyrotoxicosis (4.1%); however, in the group 60 to 69 years of age stenosis was nearly four times more frequent (in 16.5%) than in the patients with thyrotoxicosis.

CONCLUSIONS

Our studies indicate that in patients with thyrotoxicosis atherosclerosis was much less severe in the abdominal aorta and in the coronary arteries than in healthy people. This was present during comparison of groups in respect to the prevalence and area of atherosclerotic changes and the atherosclerotic index in respect to the prevalence of mild and severe degrees of atherosclerosis.

The extent of atherosclerosis in the thoracic aorta was equal in both groups.

With increasing age patients with thyrotoxicosis show a gradual intensification of atherosclerotic changes, but these develop more slowly than in healthy persons. Nevertheless, severe degrees of atherosclerosis (raised lesions occupying more than 50% of the area of a vessel), although rare, can be seen in patients with thyrotoxicosis. According to several authors, when severe atherosclerosis is found in patients with thyrotoxicosis, the duration of the disease is usually short. In these cases it is likely that thyrotoxicosis developed in the presence of severe atherosclerosis (Myasnikov and Pyatenko, 1962).

The slow development of atherosclerosis in thyrotoxicosis has been attributed by most investigators to the effect of thyroid hormones on lipid metabolism (Il'inskii, 1960; Myasnikov, 1960, 1965; Boyd, 1961; Myant, 1964; Leites, 1966; Myasnikov, 1969). In thyrotoxicosis there is a fall in blood cholesterol and its fractions and a tendency toward a decrease in total lipids and phospholipids. These data support our findings, which showed a decrease in the area with fatty streaks in all vessels in patients with thyrotoxicosis.

Patients with thyrotoxicosis not only have a smaller area with fatty streaks (compared to healthy people), but they also demonstrate a lower degree of calcification of plaques. This probably results from the disorders of calcium metabolism observed in thyrotoxicosis (Royer and Mathien, 1962; Adams *et al.*, 1967). In particular, increased activity of the thyroid gland is associated with a rise in the secretion of thyrocalcitonin, which has a hypocalcemic action (Corvilain, 1967; Care *et al.*, 1967). In addition, experimental data indicate that thyroxin may have a role in the rapid elimination of exogenous calcium (Gitters and Irvin, 1966).

The characteristic features of atherosclerosis in patients with thyrotoxicosis are probably also related to a change in the clotting system (Pavlovskii and Korvatskii, 1963; Tagi-Zade, 1967; Zaitsev and Ananchenko, 1967). In thyrotoxicosis there is a fall in the activity of the clotting system and a rise in fibrinolytic activity.

Histological study of the aorta and coronary arteries in 19 cases with thyrotoxicosis failed to reveal a single case with accumulation of fibrin on the surface of the plaques or beneath the plaques.

Thus the slow development of atherosclerosis in patients with thyrotoxicosis probably can be explained by the changes in lipid and calcium metabolism and by disorders of the clotting system, which accompany this condition.

10

Atherosclerosis and Hypertension[1]

Clarification of the role of hypertension in the development of atherosclerotic changes is of interest for the information it may provide concerning the etiology and pathogenesis of atherosclerosis, and also for the understanding it may bring of relationships between these two commonly associated diseases.

According to the epidemiological data, hypertension is an important factor in the development of ischemic heart disease. Clinical observations also demonstrate the frequent combination of hypertensive disease and atherosclerosis (Myasnikov, 1965; Kannel *et al.*, 1968; Freis, 1969; Stambler, 1971; Mitchell, 1971; Shkhvatsabaya and Metelitsa, 1971). These studies include discussions of the clinical manifestations of atherosclerosis, but the effect of hypertension on the development and course of the morphological signs of the atherosclerotic process in various parts of the arterial system is not completely clear. Robertson and Strong (1968) and Sternby (1968) established that in hypertension there is intense development of atherosclerotic lesions in the large vessels. Some investigators have failed to demonstrate any definite correlation between high blood pressure and the degree of atherosclerotic changes (Harrison and Wood, 1949; Shigeo-Okinaka, 1963; Schwartz *et al.*, 1965; Rasson and Van den Straeten, 1969).

The results of comparative macroscopic studies of atherosclerotic changes in the large arteries in patients with hypertension are not uniform. In this respect the works of Davis and Klainer (1940) are quite significant. After comparing the severity of coronary atherosclerosis in 137 hypertensive patients with controls the authors concluded that the patients with hypertension have more severe degrees of atherosclerosis than patients without hypertension. But the same authors found a low degree of atherosclerosis in patients with hypertension who died from ischemic heart disease. They also found more severe atherosclerosis in patients with normal blood pressure. From

[1] This chapter was written by E. E. Matova, D.Sc., senior scientist of the All Union Scientific Cardiological Center, Academy of Medical Sciences, USSR.

these observations they concluded that hypertension predisposes to the development of ischemic heart disease with a low degree of atherosclerosis.

HYPERTENSIVE DISEASE

To study the degree of atherosclerotic changes in hypertensive disease a morphometric study of the aorta and coronary arteries was carried out in 1,670 people from 30 to 69 years of age who died from hypertension. Of the 1,670, 1,021 were males and 649 females. A combination of hypertensive disease with ischemic heart disease was present in 70 ± 1.4% of fatal cases of hypertension in males and 49 ± 1.9% in females. Death from cerebrovascular disorders (mainly cerebral hemorrhage, rarely mixed types) occurred in 26 ± 1.3% of the males and 46 ± 1.9% of the females. In the remaining cases lesions in other organs related to atherosclerosis or renal failure (4–5% of cases) were the cause of death.

The results of visual-planimetric assessment of different types of atherosclerotic lesions (lipidosis, fibrous plaques, complicated lesions, and calcification) were compared with the corresponding values of a control group of EHI of the same age (see chapter 1).

Prevalence of Atherosclerotic Changes in the Aorta and Coronary Arteries

In the fourth decade of life in males with hypertension fibrous plaques were present in the aorta in 82% of cases, versus 56% of the cases in a control group; in the fifth decade of life in 94% and 85%, respectively; in the sixth decade in 99% and 93%, and in the seventh decade in 100% and 98%.

Thus the differences in the prevalence of fibrous plaques in the aorta were significant only in the young age group. After the age of 50 atherosclerosis is almost always present in the aorta, independent of the presence of hypertension. Similar relations are observed in females.

The prevalence of complicated lesions and calcification in hypertensive patients is considerably higher than in a control group (Table 44). The prevalence of calcification in the abdominal aorta in males over 60 years of age is an exception (68% in the hypertensive group and 64% in the control group; this difference was not statistically significant).

In the young age groups, fibrous plaques are observed more frequently in the coronary arteries than in the aorta, and their prevalence in hypertensive patients is higher than in the control group. In males, in the fourth decade of life fibrous plaques were present in 89% as compared to 71% in the control group. In the fifth decade of life the corresponding values in males were 95% and 87%, in females 87% and 68% ($p \leqslant 0.05$); in the sixth decade of life 96%

Table 44. Age-standardized Indices of Prevalence of Complicated Lesions (Co) and Calcification (Ca)

	Groups	Abdominal aorta		Left anterior descending coronary artery	
		Co	Ca	Co	Ca
Males (30–69 yrs)	1*	26.7	29.5	3.5	20.5
	2	53.5	42.0	15.2	39.5
	3	48.2	32.0	4.5	17.7
	4	53.7	43.2	22.7	58.0
	5	46.5	45.7	21.0	56.0
Females (40–60 yrs)	1	21.3	27.0	2.6	18.6
	2	44.6	49.0	10.6	30.0
	3	37.6	44.3	5.5	16.3
	4	47.6	51.3	19.0	54.0
	5	48.0	45.6	21.0	54.0

* 1, control; 2, hypertensive disease (all groups); 3, essential hypertension; 4, ischemic heart disease with hypertension; 5, ischemic heart disease with normal blood pressure.

and 93% in males and 86% and 80% in females ($p \leqslant 0.05$). Thus differences between groups with and without hypertension in the prevalence of fibrous plaques in the coronary arteries are found in patients under 50 years of age. Complicated lesions and calcification in the coronary arteries are also considerably more frequent in patients with hypertensive disease than in healthy subjects (Table 44).

Comparisons of Atherosclerotic Areas in the Aorta and Coronary Arteries

The age-related changes in the area with various types of atherosclerotic lesions in patients with hypertension duplicate the age-related changes in atherosclerosis in EHI. In each subsequent decade of life the area with fibrous plaques in the aorta was larger than in the previous one, and the area with fatty streaks decreased. Complicated lesions and calcification in the aorta appeared 10 to 20 years earlier than in subjects belonging to a control group.

In the coronary arteries there was no increase in the area with fatty streaks with age; thus the total area with atherosclerosis mainly corresponds to the area with fibrous plaques.

There was a definite increase in the area with fibrous plaques, complicated lesions, and calcification in the aorta and coronary arteries in patients with hypertension, compared to controls (Table 45). The area with fatty streaks in most age groups was larger in EHI than in patients with hypertension.

The absence of a correlation between the level of the blood pressure and the area with fatty streaks in the aorta was also noted by Mitchell *et al.* (1964), Schwartz *et al.* (1965), and Evans (1965).

It is necessary to stress, however, that during visual-planimetric assessment of the area with atherosclerotic lesions, lipids in the region of fibrous plaques were not taken into account. Therefore the quantitative estimate of lipidosis, when calculated in this manner, was limited. It can be said with certainty that the formation of fibrous plaques, complicated lesions, and calcification starts earlier and takes place more rapidly in a group with hypertension than in a control group. For example, in males dying from hypertension in the age group 30 to 39 years, the area with raised atherosclerotic lesions in the abdominal aorta was 21.6 times larger than in a group of healthy males a decade younger. In the healthy males in the same period the area with raised lesions increased only 4.5 times. The corresponding values for the coronary arteries were 8.2 (hypertension) and 3.4 (control).

The effect of the hypertensive factor on atherosclerosis is somewhat reduced with age, since the growth of atherosclerotic lesions slows. If it is assumed that the duration of hypertension did not exceed 10 years in subjects who died from hypertension aged 50 to 59 years, then the area with atherosclerosis in the aorta increased fivefold during a decade, but in healthy people only doubled during that period. In the coronary arteries the respective values were 2.6 (hypertensive disease) and 1.4 (control).

Atherosclerosis in Patients with Hypertension and in Patients in whom Atherosclerosis is the Main Disease

Since in nearly all our studies there was a combination of hypertension with ischemic disease of the heart or brain, the question arises to what extent the noticeable increase in the area with raised atherosclerotic lesions in the aorta and coronary arteries is due to hypertension alone and not to a feature of atherosclerosis in all patients, independent of hypertension.

To settle this question a comparison of atherosclerotic lesions in patients with hypertension in combination with atherosclerosis, and in patients with atherosclerosis without hypertension was conducted (see chapter 2).

There were no differences in the prevalence of fibrous plaques, calcification, and complicated lesions in the aorta noted between a group of patients with hypertension and those with atherosclerosis without hypertension.

The area of the thoracic and abdominal aorta with atherosclerotic lesions in patients with hypertensive disease was larger than in patients with athero-

Table 45. Area with Raised Atherosclerotic Lesions

Age and Sex	No. of cases			Abdominal aorta					Left anterior descending coronary artery				
	1	2	3	1* M ± SE	p	2 M ± SE	p	3 M ± SE	1 M ± SE	p	2 M ± SE	p	3 M ± SE
Males													
30–39	585	72	27	3.8 ± 0.3	×	17.3 ± 2.8	—	11.0 ± 4.1	10.5 ± 0.4	×	25.4 ± 2.7	—	22.9 ± 3.4
40–49	328	131	77	14.6 ± 0.9	×	42.2 ± 2.6	×	34.9 ± 3.6	21.1 ± 1.1	×	45.2 ± 2.5	—	51.7 ± 3.7
50–59	248	386	173	28.7 ± 1.4	×	58.4 ± 1.5	×	47.9 ± 2.3	29.5 ± 1.4	×	55.1 ± 1.5	×	49.2 ± 2.3
60–69	142	432	189	50.2 ± 2.5	×	67.7 ± 1.3	×	60.3 ± 1.7	41.7 ± 2.2	×	58.5 ± 1.4	—	59.6 ± 1.7
Females													
40–49	115	53	19	12.3 ± 1.2	×	38.1 ± 3.9	×	18.9 ± 7.6	9.7 ± 1.0	×	24.2 ± 3.8	—	28.7 ± 7.0
50–59	120	167	47	22.3 ± 1.8	×	50.5 ± 2.2	—	46.6 ± 3.5	17.8 ± 1.4	×	42.8 ± 2.2	—	40.4 ± 5.5
60–69	86	416	150	41.7 ± 3.3	×	66.9 ± 1.1	×	58.1 ± 1.9	32.9 ± 2.8	×	51.7 ± 1.3	—	54.3 ± 2.0

* M, mean area with lesion; SE, standard error; 1, control group (essentially healthy); 2, hypertensive disease (all groups); 3, atherosclerosis with hypertension (all groups); ×, differences were significant at level of $p \leqslant 0.05$; —, absence of significant differences.

sclerosis without hypertension in all the age groups studied. However, the differences were not always statistically significant (Table 45). In hypertension the area with fibrous plaques predominates. The areas with complicated lesions and calcification in the aorta did not differ significantly in the two groups.

The differences between patients with hypertension and patients with atherosclerosis without hypertension in the intensity of atherosclerosis in the coronary arteries were less pronounced than in the aorta. The prevalence of complicated lesions and calcification in the coronary arteries in a group of hypertensives and in victims of atherosclerosis who did not suffer from hypertension was the same. There was only a tendency for the area with atherosclerosis in the coronary arteries to be greater in hypertensives. This was more pronounced in the right coronary artery than in the left. Distinct differences between patients with hypertensive disease and patients with atherosclerosis with normal blood pressure were present in the area of the coronary arteries with complicated lesions and calcification.

There were no significant differences in the prevalence of stenosis of the coronary arteries between patients with hypertension (group 1) and patients with atherosclerosis as the main disease (group 2). In the fourth decade of life the prevalence of stenosis in males in the first group was 12%, in the second, 8%; in the fifth decade, 28% and 34% respectively; in the sixth decade, 46% and 45%; in the seventh, 52% and 56%. In females, in the fifth decade of life it was 4% and 18%, respectively; in the sixth, 23% and 33%; and in the seventh, 37% and 40%. The somewhat greater prevalence of stenosis in group 2 (primarily atherosclerosis) may be due to various patterns of death. In particular, there was high frequency of cerebrovascular disorders in hypertensives and a high frequency of coronary disorders in subjects dying from atherosclerosis.

Atherosclerosis, Hypertension, and Ischemic Heart Disease

In ischemic heart disease combined with hypertension, the area with atherosclerosis in the thoracic and abdominal aorta was larger than in patients with ischemic heart disease with normal blood pressure. The differences between these groups in the area with fibrous plaques, complicated lesions, and calcification were similar to those noted during an analysis of the groups with hypertension and atherosclerosis without hypertension, taken together, ignoring the cause of death. Complicated lesions and calcification in the abdominal aorta in the presence of ischemic heart disease in subjects having high blood pressure before death are seen more frequently than in subjects not suffering from hypertension (Table 44).

No significant differences were found in the prevalence of fibrous plaques, complicated lesions, calcification, or stenotic changes in coronary arteries in ischemic heart disease with hypertension and ischemic heart disease without hypertension (Tables 44 and 46).

Table 46. Prevalence of Stenosed Coronary Arteries in Ischemic Heart Disease Patients

Age and Sex	Ischemic heart disease with hypertension	*p*	Ischemic heart disease without hypertension
Males			
30–39	12.5 ± 4.4	> 0.05	8.0 ± 5.5
40–49	35.1 ± 5.0	> 0.05	32.5 ± 7.5
50–59	56.5 ± 3.0	> 0.05	52.2 ± 4.7
60–69	61.0 ± 2.9	> 0.05	61.5 ± 3.7

Patients with ischemic heart disease with hypertension showed a greater area of atherosclerotic changes in the right coronary artery and the left circumflex coronary artery than patients with ischemic heart disease with normal blood pressure. In the left anterior descending coronary artery the differences between these groups were less pronounced than in the other coronary arteries. In hypertensive disease it is mainly the area with fibrous plaques that increases in the coronary arteries; the differences in the areas with complicated lesions and calcification were quite variable.

In ischemic heart disease the intensity of the atherosclerotic process in the coronary arteries was slightly dependent on the presence of hypertension.

SECONDARY RENAL HYPERTENSION

Evidence for the accelerating effect of secondary hypertension on the development of atherosclerotic changes was obtained mainly from experimental hypertension (Deming, 1966). Experimental hypertension is pathogenetically closer to the various forms of secondary hypertension in man than to essential hypertension. The results of these experimental studies support the atherogenic effect of the hypertensive syndrome, but contradict clinical practice, because atherosclerosis causing ischemic heart disease is rarely seen in patients with secondary, particularly renal, hypertension (Hamburger *et al.*, 1965; Kononyachenko, 1971; Ratner, 1971). It is possible that azotemic states have an inhibitory effect on the development of atherosclerosis (Myasnikov, 1965), but this hypothesis is not yet supported by adequate data.

There are relatively few reports in the literature on the nature of atherosclerotic changes in the aorta and coronary arteries in patients with secondary hypertension, and these are based on a small number of observations (Steiner and Domanski, 1942; Fishberg, 1944; Rau, 1956; Maher and Schreier, 1957; Sacks, 1960).

We studied the atherosclerotic changes in the aorta and coronary arteries in 384 patients with renal disease and hypertension (chronic glomerulonephritis, chronic pyelonephritis) who died at ages from 10 to 69 years. All the comparisons were done in identical conditions and were grouped by decade of life.

Prevalence of Atherosclerotic Changes in the Aorta and Coronary Arteries

Atherosclerotic changes in the aorta and coronary arteries in secondary hypertension are already present in childhood. Fibrous plaques were seen in the aorta in half of the cases in children 10 to 19 years of age. In the age group 20 to 29 fibrous plaques in the aorta were three times more frequent (63 %) in cases with hypertension than in the control group (20 %); from 30 to 39 years, in 92 % of the cases with hypertension as compared to 56 % in the control group. Fibrous plaques were present in the coronary arteries of males between 20 and 29 years in $73 \pm 7.2\%$ of patients with hypertension versus in 49 % of the controls. In the fourth decade of life the prevalence of fibrous plaques in secondary hypertension was 97 %, which considerably exceeded the values in the control group (71 %). The prevalence of complicated lesions and calcification in the aorta and coronary arteries is presented in Table 44.

Area of the Aorta and Coronary Arteries with Atherosclerotic Changes

Patients with secondary hypertension show a greater prevalence of fibrous plaques and a greater area of altered intimal surface in the aorta than do EHI. In males 20 to 29 years old the area with fibrous plaques in the abdominal aorta in secondary hypertensives was $14 \pm 3.6\%$ of the intimal surface versus only $0.8 \pm 0.1\%$ in EH males of the same age group ($p < 0.01$); in females the values were $19.2 \pm 4.1\%$ and $0.9 \pm 0.3\%$, respectively ($p < 0.01$). The total area of the aorta occupied by atherosclerotic changes is greater in patients with secondary hypertension than in healthy people, in all the age groups up to 69 years, both in males and in females (Table 47). Fatty streaks are the exception; they occupy a larger area in the aorta of essentially healthy people as compared to patients with hypertension.

The total area of the coronary arteries with atherosclerotic changes was also considerably greater in patients with hypertension than in EHI, in almost all age groups. These differences between patients with hypertension and

Table 47. Area with Raised Atherosclerotic Lesions

Age and Sex	No. of cases			Abdominal aorta					Left anterior descending coronary artery				
	1	2	3	1* M ± SE	p	2 M ± SE	p	3 M ± SE	1 M ± SE	p	2 M ± SE	p	3 M ± SE
Males													
20–29	505	37	0	0.8 ± 0.1	×	14.0 ± 3.7			3.1 ± 0.2	×	17.2 ± 3.5		
30–39	585	49	72	3.8 ± 0.3	×	33.5 ± 3.8	×	17.3 ± 2.8	10.5 ± 0.4	×	34.0 ± 3.0	×	25.4 ± 2.7
40–49	328	49	131	14.6 ± 0.9	×	38.7 ± 3.9	—	42.2 ± 2.6	21.2 ± 1.1	×	35.5 ± 4.1	×	45.2 ± 2.5
50–59	248	30	386	28.7 ± 1.4	×	55.5 ± 6.0	—	58.4 ± 1.5	29.4 ± 1.4	—	34.6 ± 5.0	×	55.1 ± 1.5
60–69	142	22	432	50.2 ± 2.5	×	66.0 ± 5.6	—	67.7 ± 1.3	41.7 ± 2.2	×	54.5 ± 5.5	—	58.5 ± 1.4
Females													
20–29	109	24	0	0.9 ± 0.3	×	19.2 ± 4.1			1.9 ± 0.4	×	10.8 ± 3.1		
30–39	125	26	13	2.9 ± 0.4	×	22.7 ± 5.6	—	31.6 ± 8.1	5.5 ± 0.7	×	20.5 ± 5.4	—	18.2 ± 5.6
40–49	115	39	53	12.3 ± 1.2	×	41.9 ± 4.4	—	38.1 ± 3.9	9.7 ± 1.0	×	32.0 ± 5.3	—	24.2 ± 3.8
50–59	120	41	167	22.3 ± 1.8	×	54.6 ± 5.2	—	50.5 ± 2.2	17.8 ± 1.8	×	27.6 ± 4.1	×	42.8 ± 2.2
60–69	86	46	416	41.7 ± 3.3	×	65.9 ± 4.2	—	66.9 ± 1.1	32.8 ± 2.8	×	47.7 ± 4.7	—	51.7 ± 1.3

* M, mean area with lesion; SE, standard error; 1, control group (essentially healthy); 2, secondary hypertension; 3, essential hypertension; ×, differences were significant at a level of $p \leqslant 0.05$; —, absence of significant differences.

controls result mainly from differences in the area with fibrous plaques. The areas with complicated lesions and calcification in the coronary arteries were similar in the patients with hypertension and in EHI. In elderly males calcification in the coronary arteries of hypertensive patients occupied an even smaller area than in males in the control group ($p < 0.05$).

Atherosclerotic Changes in Secondary and Essential Hypertension

A comparison of atherosclerotic changes in secondary hypertension and in essential hypertension demonstrated that in the fourth decade of life the area of atherosclerotic changes in the thoracic and abdominal aorta of males was twice as great in patients with secondary hypertension as in patients with essential hypertension; over 40 years of age there was a similar degree of advanced atherosclerosis in the aorta in both groups (Table 47).

Atherosclerotic changes in the coronary arteries of males below 40 years of age with secondary hypertension occupy a greater area than in patients with essential hypertension. Thus the increase in the area of atherosclerotic changes caused by hypertension is independent of the etiology of the hypertension. This agrees with the experimental and clinical data indicating that hypertensive states of varying etiology share many biochemical and humoral values. The changes in the vessel walls, in particular the increased permeability of the vessel, have been found to be similar in both types of hypertension (Kasatkina, 1969; Myasnikov *et al.*, 1971).

Atherosclerotic Changes in Secondary Hypertension and Ischemic Heart Disease

It has been questioned whether renal hypertension produces morphological differences in coronary atherosclerosis, since these cases do not commonly have clinical or morphological findings of acute or chronic coronary insufficiency.

We attempted to answer this question by comparing the features of atherosclerotic changes in the coronary arteries in patients with renal hypertension with the features of atherosclerosis in patients with ischemic heart disease and normal blood pressure.

In the young age group atherosclerotic changes in the coronary arteries in patients with renal hypertension occupy an even greater area than in subjects of the same age dying from ischemic heart disease. In males of 30 to 39 years of age with renal hypertension the area with atherosclerotic changes in the right coronary artery was 35 $\pm$ 4.0; in the left circumflex coronary artery, 31 $\pm$ 3.9%; in the left anterior descending coronary artery, 37 $\pm$ 3.9%. In ischemic heart disease the corresponding values were 17 $\pm$ 4.0%, 16 $\pm$ 3.4%, and 25 $\pm$ 3.3% ($p < 0.05$). In the group 40 to 49 years of age, in both males and females, atherosclerotic changes occupied similar areas in the coronary arteries in patients with renal hypertension and in patients with ischemic heart disease. In subjects over 50 years of age the area of the coronary arteries with atherosclerotic changes was greater in the group with ischemic heart disease. Atherosclerotic changes in the coronary arteries in renal hypertension, particularly in the young age group, have certain characteristics: (1) fewer complicated lesions and less calcification (Table 44); (2) no correlation between the area of atherosclerotic changes in the coronary arteries and the area with calcification; and (3) rare development of stenosis. Below 50 years of age stenosis in renal hypertension was found only in isolated cases, in spite of the marked prevalence of fibrous plaques in the intima of the coronary arteries. In contrast, in young subjects dying from myocardial infarction, with the same area of fibrous plaques, severe stenosis of the coronary arteries was observed in 54% of cases.

Stenosis of the coronary arteries was noted more frequently in old and elderly subjects with renal hypertension than in the young, but remained less frequent than in patients with ischemic heart disease. Thus the lack of symptoms from coronary atherosclerosis with renal hypertension probably results from the absence of coronary stenosis and the presence of fibrous atherosclerotic plaques.

In our patients with renal hypertension there were as a rule no morphological signs of acute or chronic coronary insufficiency, nor were there focal changes in the myocardium. We did not observe a single fatal case of myocardial infarction in combination with symptomatic renal hypertension in the patients below 50 years of age. Only two cases of myocardial infarction were present in males over 50 years of age (3.8% of the males in this age group). In the myocardium of patients with symptomatic renal hypertension post-infarction scars were noted in only one male and one female in the age group over 60.

CONCLUSIONS

In all types of arterial hypertension conditions are created that favor the progression of fibrous atherosclerotic plaques. The atherogenic effect of hypertension appears more distinctly in the young. The differences in the degree of atherosclerotic changes in patients with normal and high blood pressure diminish with age.

There is a possibility that hypertension in older individuals, i.e., essential hypertension, is a secondary sclerotic hypertension which appears in patients with atherosclerosis. Increased rigidity of the aorta, lesions in the baroreceptor apparatus, atherosclerotic occlusion of the renal arteries, and cerebral atherosclerosis have some role in its pathogenesis. In elderly people with sclerotic hypertension atherosclerotic changes in the coronary arteries may already be so pronounced that the effect of hypertension on their progression is of little importance.

An important factor which may, to a considerable extent, determine the intensity of the atherogenic effect of hypertension is the chronological sequence of the development of hypertensive disease and atherosclerosis. Different chronological variations in the sequence of formation of these combined diseases may, to a considerable extent, explain the variability of atherosclerotic changes in patients with hypertension.

The effect of hypertension on the development of atherosclerotic changes is not uniform in different vessels. The atherogenic effect of different types of hypertension is more distinct in the aorta than in coronary arteries.

The development of atherosclerotic changes is basically the same in patients with essential hypertension and in patients with secondary renal hypertension. In both the area with fibrous atherosclerotic plaques expands more rapidly. There is no distinct relationship between hypertension and the development of complicated lesions in the region of fibrous plaques (erosion, intimal hemorrhages, thromboses), or with stenosis of the lumen of the coronary arteries. Changes of this type are characteristic for ischemic heart disease regardless of the presence of normal or high blood pressure.

Conclusion

At the present time diseases produced by atherosclerotic lesions of the arteries of the heart, brain, and lower extremities are frequent. These diseases are the primary cause of death of the adult population in many countries. A large number of studies show a rise in the frequency of diseases caused by atherosclerosis not only in people of middle and old age but also in the young. The above situation justifies intensive study of the clinical, morphological, biochemical, and epidemiological aspects of atherosclerosis.

In the study of atherosclerosis it should be remembered that the development of the atherosclerotic process in man continues throughout his life. The biochemical and clinical manifestations of atherosclerosis, particularly in the early stages of the disease, are not constant. This may explain the discrepancy between the degree of atherosclerosis found at autopsy and that encountered in living subjects with the clinical manifestations of the disease. Some cases are seen with severe atherosclerosis of the aorta and coronary arteries without any clinical signs of the disease. Alternatively, there are cases in which myocardial infarction resulted from thrombosis of a coronary artery that occurred in an isolated atherosclerotic plaque with an erosion.

Therefore, only morphological investigations can give authentic results of the prevalence of atherosclerosis and the degree of its development in subjects belonging to certain groups or populations. This applies uniformly to the study of the effect of various diseases on the atherosclerotic process.

The comparative studies we conducted revealed the characteristics of the atherosclerotic process in certain groups of people depending on various conditions. In this connection major credit should be given to the work of the study group of histopathologists from various countries, who, on the initiative of the World Health Organization, developed the methodological basis for performing an epidemiological study of atherosclerosis with the use of pathological specimens. The use of a unified terminology and classification of atherosclerotic lesions and methods of clinical assessment permits us to characterize the changes in the vessels objectively and to obtain data suitable for comparative investigations.

In the present work a morphometric study was conducted of the degree of atherosclerotic change in the vessels of patients with diabetes mellitus, malignant tumors, cirrhosis of the liver, rheumatic heart disease, chronic lung disease, chronic pulmonary tuberculosis, thyrotoxicosis and hypertension. In this study, all the cases with a combination of one disease with another were excluded from analysis. Therefore we were able to study the effect of various diseases as free as possible from the contributions of other diseases.

This study reveals qualitative and quantitative differences in the rate of development of atherosclerosis in different diseases (Figs. 32, 33).

In diabetic patients the acceleration of atherosclerosis was clearly age-dependent. Below age 50 the degree of atherosclerosis in most vessels (89.7%) was the same as in healthy people. However, in patients over 50 years of age atherosclerosis in the aorta and coronary arteries considerably exceeded that in healthy people and differed little in degree from those who died from the complications of atherosclerosis. From these data it could be concluded that diabetes as such does not significantly affect the development of atherosclerosis, and that the combination of diabetes with severe atherosclerosis is probably not due to the rapid development of atherosclerosis under the influence of diabetes. On the contrary, it may be that the development of diabetes results from severe atherosclerosis; more precisely, it is possible that atherosclerosis may be an important predisposing factor to the development of diabetes through involvement of the arteries that supply the blood to the pancreas gland, in particular the branches of the splenic artery.

At the same time, the data presented do not exclude the possible effect of diabetes mellitus on the development of atherosclerosis, particularly in the young. However, at the present time appropriate and early treatment of diabetes is generally given and may, to some extent, neutralize the effect of diabetes on atherosclerosis. Sedov also pointed out the possible inhibitory effect of the modern treatment of diabetes on the development of atherosclerosis. Together with us he performed an epidemiological study of atherosclerosis in autopsy specimens of subjects who died in the city of Irkutsk. In addition, a study of analogous materials from five European cities[1] failed to demonstrate any significant difference in the degree of atherosclerosis in diabetic patients treated with insulin or diet and those treated with oral hypoglycemic agents. It is true that these studies were conducted mainly in subjects over 50 years of age.

Cases with a combination of diabetes mellitus and hypertension demonstrated the most severe atherosclerotic changes. However, in these cases the degree of atherosclerosis was only slightly greater than in patients with hypertension without diabetes mellitus.

Patients with malignant tumors of all types showed no significant difference in the degree of atherosclerosis as compared with EHI. There was only a tendency toward less pronounced changes in the coronary arteries in patients

[1] The WHO study in Tallin, Ryazan, Yalta (USSR), Prague (Czechoslovakia) and Malmö (Sweden).

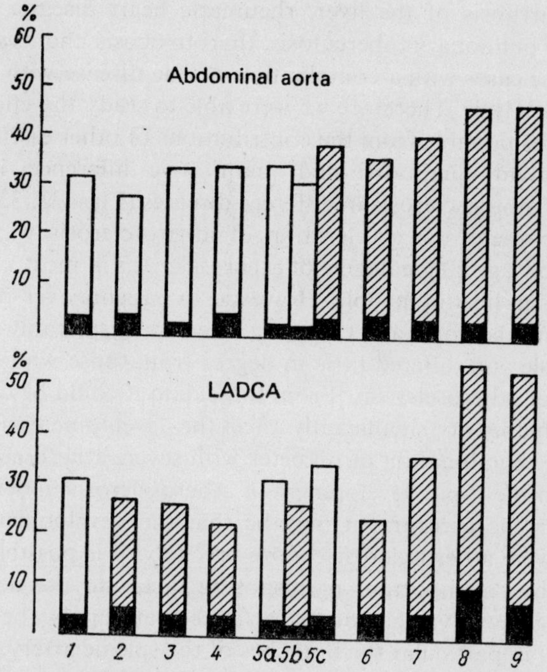

Figure 32. Age-standardized (40–69 years) indices of the area of raised lesions in males with various diseases. *1*, healthy; *2*, cirrhosis of the liver; *3*, pulmonary tuberculosis; *4*, chronic lung diseases; *5a*, malignant tumors (all forms); *5b*, gastric carcinoma; *5c*, carcinoma of the lungs; *6*, rheumatic heart disease; *7*, diabetes mellitus not associated with hypertension; *8*, diabetes mellitus associated with hypertension; *9*, atherosclerosis as the principal disease. The solid part of the columns indicate the area with calcification; the lined part of the columns indicate that the differences in raised lesions are statistically significant when compared with a group of healthy people (*1*) in respect to area ($p \leqslant 0.05$); the clear area of the columns indicates the absence of statistically significant difference from a group of healthy people. The ordinate shows the changed area as percentage of the intimal surface of the vessel.

with malignant tumors. There were no differences in the degree of atherosclerosis in the aorta of emaciated and nonemaciated patients with malignant tumors. In the coronary arteries, however, the nonemaciated patients tended to show greater changes.

Analysis of the degree of atherosclerosis in patients with malignant tumors in all the groups can mask unique features of the development of atherosclerosis in carcinomas of various types. In males with carcinoma of the lungs the degree of atherosclerosis in the aorta and coronary arteries was considerably

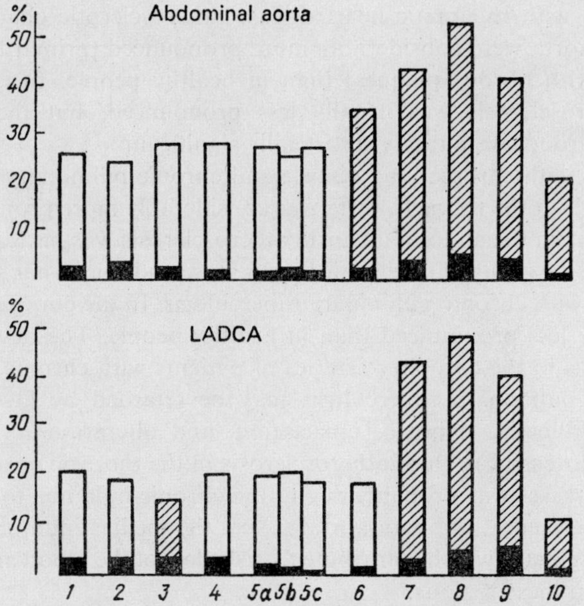

Figure 33. Age-standardized (40–69 years) indices of the area with raised lesions in females with various diseases. *5c*, carcinoma of the breast; *10*, thyrotoxicosis. Remainder of the legends are the same as in Fig. 32.

greater than in patients with gastric carcinoma, and somewhat greater than in EHI. Similarly, some differences were found in the degree of atherosclerosis in carcinoma of the ovaries, the uterus, and the breast in females. In patients with carcinoma of the ovaries, particularly in the fifth decade of life, atherosclerosis was more marked than in a control group of healthy females; in patients with carcinoma of the breast or uterus there were inverse relationships. These features of the development of atherosclerosis in females with carcinoma of the ovaries and breast show the importance of endocrine factors in the development of atherosclerosis. In females with carcinoma of the ovaries (the majority had a history of ophorectomy) the antiatherosclerotic effect of estrogen is reduced because of decreased synthesis of estrogen; in patients with carcinoma of the breast this effect is intensified.

In patients with cirrhosis of the liver the area of atherosclerotic changes in the aorta differed little from the changes in EHI. In patients with cirrhosis coronary atherosclerosis was usually considerably less pronounced than in EHI. The unusual feature of atherosclerosis in patients with cirrhosis of the liver is the considerably smaller area with lipidosis; in contrast, calcification of the aorta and coronary arteries in patients with cirrhosis of the liver was seen frequently and was more extensive than in healthy people.

In patients with rheumatic heart disease atherosclerotic changes in both parts of the aorta were considerably more pronounced (primarily due to the larger area with fibrous plaques) than in healthy people. In the coronary arteries atherosclerosis was usually less pronounced, but the differences between the groups were rarely statistically significant.

In patients with chronic lung disease and chronic pulmonary tuberculosis atherosclerosis in the thoracic aorta was considerably more pronounced than in the healthy; in the abdominal aorta atherosclerosis was basically the same as controls in the group with chronic lung disease and somewhat more marked in the group with chronic pulmonary tuberculosis. In the coronary arteries it was as a rule less pronounced than in healthy people. The development of atherosclerosis in the coronary arteries of patients with chronic lung disease and chronic pulmonary tuberculosis may be retarded by factors such as hypocholesterolemia, hypoxia, emaciation, and alteration in the clotting system. The intensification of atherosclerosis in the thoracic aorta in patients with these diseases was probably due to the chronic inflammatory process in the lungs, the pleura, the para-aortal tissue, the mediastinum and the para-aortic lymph glands, which contribute to disorders of the blood and lymphatic circulations in these regions.

In patients with thyrotoxicosis atherosclerosis in the abdominal aorta and coronary arteries was considerably less severe than in healthy subjects; atherosclerosis was basically the same in both groups in the thoracic aorta.

In hypertension the formation of fibrous plaques in the aorta and coronary arteries is accelerated, while the rate of development of lipidosis does not change significantly.

In secondary renal hypertension in patients with chronic glomerulonephritis and pyelonephritis there is also accelerated development of atherosclerotic changes in the aorta and coronary arteries. In young subjects with renal hypertension the degree of atherosclerosis in the aorta and coronary arteries was much greater than in patients with essential hypertension.

In renal hypertension there is accelerated development of smooth atherosclerotic plaques in the coronary arteries. These occupy a considerable part of the intimal surface, but they do not usually undergo ulceration, calcification, or thrombosis. The development of coronary stenosis is rare in these patients, which explains their asymptomatic course.

The accelerating effect of arterial hypertension on the development of atherosclerosis in the aorta and coronary arteries was most pronounced in the young age group. The effect of arterial hypertension of different etiology on the development of atherosclerotic changes appears to be more marked in the aorta than in the coronary arteries.

The results of our study convincingly demonstrate that the development of atherosclerotic changes in the aorta and coronary arteries varies in different disease states. The effect of the diseases on the development of atherosclerosis varied in different vessels. Inhibitory factors such as hypocholesterolemia and other changes in lipid metabolism, hypotension, hypoxia, and decreased clotting were most active in retarding the development of atherosclerosis in the coronary arteries. This was observed to a varying extent with malignant tumors, cirrhosis of the liver, rheumatic heart disease, chronic lung disease, pulmonary tuberculosis, and thyrotoxicosis.

The degree of atherosclerosis in the aorta in these diseases (with the exception of thyrotoxicosis) was the same or greater than that observed in EHI. It should be noted, however, that in the diseases associated with hypocholesterolemia the area with fatty streaks was smaller not only in the coronary arteries but also in the aorta. The effect of hypocholesterolemia on the development of fibrous plaques in the aorta and coronary arteries was less distinct and not uniform. In the coronary arteries, in addition to the decrease in the area with lipidosis there was also a definite tendency toward a decrease in the area with fibrous plaques, i.e., there was suppression of the development of fibrous plaques. However, in the aorta suppression of the development of fibrous plaques was noted only in patients with thyrotoxicosis.

The extent of the area with calcification is usually directly dependent on the age and the degree of other types of atherosclerotic changes, which are mainly fibrous plaques. However, in patients with cirrhosis of the liver, and to a lesser extent in patients with chronic lung disease and pulmonary tuberculosis, there is a greater tendency toward accumulation of calcium in atherosclerotic plaques. This is indicated not only from data showing the area with calcification but also by the ratio of the area with fibrous plaques to the area with calcification. In the above diseases each percent of the area with calcification (particularly in the coronary arteries) corresponds to a smaller area with fibrous plaques in healthy people.

The rates of development of atherosclerosis are not the same in different vessels. This has been observed both in a group of EHI and in patients dying from various diseases. In a number of diseases (particularly rheumatic heart disease, chronic lung disease, and pulmonary tuberculosis) considerable differences were found in the degree of atherosclerosis compared with a group of EHI.

In respect to the degree of atherosclerosis in the coronary arteries (total area with raised lesions) the effects may be summarized (Figs. 32 and 33). The changes were the least extensive in patients with thyrotoxicosis.

In patients with chronic pulmonary tuberculosis and chronic lung disease the changes were always less severe than in healthy people; in most comparisons the differences between the groups were statistically significant.

In patients with cirrhosis of the liver the changes were less than in EHI; in approximately half of the comparisons the differences between the groups were found to be statistically significant.

In patients with rheumatic heart disease the changes were usually less than in EHI, but the differences were rarely statistically significant.

In patients with malignant tumors and patients with diabetes mellitus less than 50 years of age there were no significant differences as compared to changes in a group of EHI.

In patients with essential and secondary hypertension the changes were always more marked than in EHI.

In diabetic patients over age 50 the changes were always more marked than in EHI.

Of all the diseases studied only diabetes mellitus in patients over 50 and hypertension were associated with atherosclerotic changes of the same degree or greater than those found in patients dying from the various complications of atherosclerosis. In all the remaining diseases atherosclerotic changes were always considerably less marked than in patients dying from the complications of atherosclerosis. The differences were greatest in the more advanced stages of atherosclerosis—fibrous plaques, complicated lesions, and calcification.

The results of this study indicate that atherosclerosis in subjects with various diseases has different rates of development and different qualitative characteristics. The qualitative changes are variations in the individual types of lesions—fatty streaks, fibrous plaques, complicated lesions, and calcification. In all probability the effect of various diseases on the course of the atherosclerotic process in different diseases stems not from any single factor but from several factors that are characteristic for each disease. The great variations in the degree of atherosclerotic process in the groups of patients studied resulted not only from the diseases studied, but also from other factors such as professional activity, which were not analyzed in the present study. It is beyond doubt that in man atherosclerosis is a multifactorial illness. For this reason the totality of the factors which could affect atherosclerosis should be studied. Many authors have emphasized the importance of the various phases of life in the development of atherosclerosis. Davydovskii (1967) wrote that species, individual, genetic, and ecological factors, and the mode of life and its duration are responsible for the great variations in the morphological and clinical manifestations of atherosclerosis.

In the present work it has been shown that the degree of atherosclerosis is dependent on the age, sex, specific disease, and endocrine status. The results we obtained raise a series of questions which are difficult to answer.

Recent data on the pathogenesis of atherosclerosis indicate that the disease may result not only from disorders of lipid metabolism and accumulation of lipids in the intima, but also from other mechanisms (changes in hemodynamics, age, alterations in permeability and activity of the enzymes in the vessel wall, changes in its elastic character, neurogenic factors, and changes in the coagulation and anticoagulation processes). It is clear that the term "atherosclerosis" introduced in the early part of this century by Marchand characterizes only part of the change in the vascular wall, and this change may not occur at the initiation of the process. The older term "arteriosclerosis" is perhaps more suitable for describing the above mentioned changes in the vessels.

For more than 60 years disorders of cholesterol metabolism have been considered as the primary cause of atherosclerosis. The cholesterol theory of atherosclerosis which accompanied the experimental study of cholesterol-induced atherosclerosis (or, more correctly, cholesterosis of the arteries, obtained in rabbits by feeding them large doses of cholesterol) has undergone some changes and modifications, but its principle remains unchanged. The following scheme of the pathogenesis of atherosclerosis in man is acceptable even today: fatty streaks ⟶ fibrous plaques ⟶ complicated lesions, calcification.

In the metabolic theory of atherosclerosis, changes in the arterial wall are neglected; more attention is paid to the size of the lipid molecules and the ratios of various types of serum lipids, such as the ratio of cholesterol to phospholipids. Recently, according to Fredrickson, the different types of hyperlipoproteinemias have been considered to be the most important factors. Only types IIA and IV are associated with atherogenesis. If the serum cholesterol level is elevated, or if the ratio of lipids is changed or certain types of lipids are present, the conditions necessary for the initiation of atherosclerosis are present.

In spite of extensive study of this problem over the past decades, few practical results have been achieved in either prevention or treatment of atherosclerosis. On the contrary, we now face a growing epidemic of atherosclerosis.

Further, it is not completely clear that uncomplicated lipidosis (fatty streaks) should be considered as the beginning of the atherosclerotic process. This may be answered either positively or negatively, but both answers lead to several new questions that are also difficult to answer. If the answer is yes, then it must be recognized that 100% of children of both sexes in the age group 10 to 14 years have the early signs of atherosclerosis in the aorta and 50 to 60% have such signs in the coronary arteries. Fatty streaks frequently occupy 30 to 60% of the intimal surface of the aorta. Therefore it must be concluded that atherosclerosis starts before the age of 10 and that all children at present suffer from a disorder of lipid metabolism. Since it is difficult to agree with this, the thesis is advanced that to some degree the fatty streaks are reversible and that lipidosis to a certain extent is a physiological phenomenon. However, no physiological or pathological criteria for lipidosis have been advanced, nor is it clear why fatty streaks in some cases are reversible, while in others there is fibrous transformation even in childhood. In addition, even with extensive lipidosis (for example, in cases in which the area with lipidosis is 60% of the intimal surface of the aorta) the fibrous plaques are always restricted in nature and occupy not more than 2 to 5% of the intimal area of a vessel. Fibrous plaques are never diffuse in character.

There is no direct relationship between the degree of lipidosis and the development of fibrous plaques. This has been observed both in our studies and in those of others. The average area of the aorta with lipidosis in all groups studied gradually decreases after the third or fourth decade of life. However, there is not a parallel decrease in the area with fibrous plaques. In the coronary arteries the area with lipidosis changes little with age, but the area with fibrous plaques increases steadily with each decade. Similarly, in females the area with lipidosis is as a rule larger than in males, whose fibrous plaques appear earlier and develop at faster rates.

The development of a fibrous plaque at the site of a fatty streak is related not only to the presence of lipids in the vessel intima but also to the factors that determine the fate of these lipids (lipolytic activity, permeability of the vessel wall, composition of the plasma, and other factors).

Thus the data available do not support the unconditional acceptance of the above mentioned sequence for the pathogenesis of atherosclerosis. The first half of the hypothesis (lipidosis ⟶ fibrous plaque) must be reconsidered. During the last few years other possible causes for the development of fibrous plaques, and the changes predisposing to the development of the atherosclerotic process, have been studied in detail. In other words, attention has now been directed to what Myasnikov (1965) aptly termed the prelipid stage of atherosclerosis. It is clear that atherosclerotic fibrous plaques are caused not only by disorders of lipid metabolism but also by other conditions (microcirculatory disorders of the vessel wall, hyperplastic processes in the intima, hemodynamic forces, etc.). These primary changes may occur in the early stage of the process in childhood, in the young, and in the middle-aged (Zhdanov *et al.*, 1973).

The data presented in this work demonstrate the close relationship between atherosclerosis and age. As is well known, Davydovskii (1967) did not consider atherosclerosis as a disease but as a gerontological problem—a phenomenon of biological involution and aging of the body. Attention is drawn to the fact that the difference between the vessels in the degree of atherosclerosis that exists in the second or third decade of life is usually preserved throughout life. This primarily indicates the importance of local factors in the development of the atherosclerotic process.

When discussing the close relationship of atherosclerosis to age it must be noted that the process starts in the young; by 10–14 years of age 5% of children have fibrous plaques, although they occupy less than 5% of the intimal surface. By the ages 15 to 19 fibrous plaques are present in 16% of cases. The area rises considerably, so that by 30 years of age the plaques are found in 33% of cases and by 40 years of age in 65% of male deaths. These findings contradict the hypothesis that atherosclerosis is a problem of the elderly, that it is an involution problem of the aged, or that it is due to biological aging. On the contrary, they show that atherosclerosis is related to youth and even childhood, since the atherosclerotic process is started in the early phase of life.

Although aging is of great significance in the development of atherosclerosis, our data do not support the view that atherosclerosis is due to aging. Our data do not indicate that atherosclerosis is a consequence of aging rather than a disease. The data showed an extreme variation in the degree of atherosclerosis in people belonging to the same age group. Severe atherosclerotic changes were seen in some individuals in the fourth decade of life. Atherosclerotic changes are completely absent or minimal in 1 to 2% of people in the eighth and ninth decades of life. In some cases atherosclerotic lesions are not uniformly distributed in the arterial system, particularly in young subjects (primary lesions of the coronary arteries or even of a single coronary artery or cerebral artery). Also the pathological changes are not the changes characteristic of a certain age. The appearance of fibrous plaques in the aorta and even in the coronary arteries in a small number of individuals under 20 similarly shows that the process is due to a disease and not to changes in the vascular system associated with the aging. In a number of cases this disease starts at a very young age. An important task for modern medicine is to explain why younger people are being drawn into the epidemic of atherosclerosis. It is beyond doubt that aging and atherosclerosis are intimately connected, but at present it is also very clear that atherosclerosis is also connected with youth.

It remains difficult to understand the relationship between several diseases and the development of atherosclerosis. Why, in a number of diseases having relatively short duration (for example, in patients with malignant tumors), is atherosclerosis, even in the 60 to 79 year age group, of the same degree as in healthy people? These subjects usually show no clinical signs of atherosclerosis, such as myocardial infarction, vascular disorders, or gangrene of the extremities. In the age group 60 to 70 these diseases are responsible for 30 to 40% of deaths, but in patients with malignant neoplasms they are absent in a large number of cases. Atherosclerosis in the latter is usually less pronounced, and as a rule there are no signs of diseases found at autopsy (old myocardial scars, cerebral cysts, etc.). How are we to explain the role of a malignant neoplasm, which an elderly patient has for his last three to five years, in the prevention of the atherosclerotic process over his entire life? It is possible that there are some differences between patients dying from the complications of atherosclerosis and from malignant neoplasms, regarding the life styles, genetic background, and other factors. However, there are no data supporting such a hypothesis.

It is also important to note that the rates of development of atherosclerosis throughout life in different individuals are not uniform. The slow, gradual development of atherosclerosis frequently noted in healthy individuals may, in some phase of life, accelerate for unknown reasons and produce clinically apparent disease. Therefore it is possible that subjects dying from the complications of atherosclerosis, in the age group 70 to 79, had the same degree of atherosclerosis as healthy people during most of their life, and only during the last 10 to 15 years was the process accelerated, leading to the development of clinical symptoms.

Not only will many of our impressions of atherosclerosis, its etiology and pathogenesis, have to be reviewed in the course of time, but the established facts must be re-examined as well. The problem of atherosclerosis requires a new approach free from time-honored concepts and the cholesterol theory. The focus of investigations should be shifted to study of the vessel wall itself.

References

Abaeva, V. V. 1967. Revmatizm i tireotoksikoz (Rheumatic heart disease and thyrotoxicosis). Abstract of candidate thesis, Rostov-on-Don.

Abdullaev, R. A., S. A. Akhmedov, and B. Yu. Yuldashev. 1974. O razvitii ateroskleroza u bol'nykh khronicheskim gepatitom i tsirrozom pecheni. (The development of atherosclerosis in patients with chronic hepatitis and cirrhosis of the liver). *Med. zh. Uzbekistana* 1:40.

Abramova. A. A. 1967. Osobennosti izmenenii sosudov nizhnikh konechnostei pri ateroskleroticheskoi i diabeticheskoi gangrene (Vascular changes in the lower extremities in atherosclerosis and diabetic gangrene). *Trudy 4-go Vsesoyuzn. S"ezda patologoanatomov*, Moscow, p. 323.

Abrikosov, A. I., and A. I. Strukov. 1961. *Patologicheskaya anatomiya* (*Pathological anatomy*). Medgiz, Moscow, 559 p.

Ackerman, R. F., T. J. Dry, and J. E. Edwards. 1950. Relationship of various factors to the degree of coronary atherosclerosis in women. *Circulation* 1:1345.

Adams, P. H., J. Jowsey, P. J. Keley, B. I. Riggs, V. R. Kinney, and J. D. Jones. 1967. Effects of hyperthyroidism on bone and mineral metabolism in man. *Quart. J. Med.* 36:1.

Akhmetzyanov, A. A. 1967. Ateroskleroz pri khronicheskom legochnom tuberkuleze (Atherosclerosis in chronic pulmonary tuberculosis). Abstract of candidate thesis, Kazan'.

Aleksandrov, N. G. 1973. Patologicheskaya anatomiya nekotorykh endokrinnykh zhelez i dinamika ateroskleroticheskogo protsessa pri razlichnykh formakh endemicheskogo zoba (The pathological anatomy of some endocrine glands and the dynamics of the atherosclerotic process in various types of endemic goiter). Abstract of doctoral thesis, Moscow.

Alekseev, V. P. 1968. Kharakteristika ateroskleroza po sektsionnomu materialu Yakutska (The characteristics of atherosclerosis in autopsy material from Yakutsk). *Kardiologiya* 2:58.

Alekseeva, L. F. 1966. Kharakteristika ateroskleroza u bol'nykh tuberkulezom (The characteristics of atherosclerosis in tuberculous patients). *Materialy 9-i nauchn, sessii med. f-ta Yakutsk Gos. un-ta*, Yakutsk, p. 85.

Alikhanova, Z. E. 1968. Ateroskleroz pri emfizeme legkikh (Atherosclerosis in pulmonary emphysema). *Azerbaidzhansk. Med. zh.* 2:20.

Altland, P., and B. Higman. 1960. Effects of high altitude on cholesterol-fed rabbits. *Arch. Path.* 70:349.

Anestiadi, V. Kh. 1967. Ateroskleroz arterii; *Ul'trafioletovoe fotografirovanie, lyuminestsentyi i gistokhim, analizy* (Atherosclerosis of the arteries, in *Ultraviolet photography, luminescence and histochemical analysis*). *Kartya moldovenyaske*, Kishinev, 160 p.

Anichkov, N. N. 1935. Patologicheskaya anatomiya i patogenez ateroskleroza po dannym mezhdunarodnogo sektsionnogo materiala (Pathological anatomy and pathogenesis of atherosclerosis according to data from autopsy material). *Arkh. biol. nauk* 1:51.

Anichkov, N. H. 1947. Sosudy (The vessels), in *Chastnaya patologicheskaya anatomiya* (*Pathological anatomy*), A. I. Abrikosov, ed., 2nd ed. Moscow, 574 p.

Armstrong, H. G., and J. W. Heim. 1938. The effect of repeated daily exposure to anoxemia. *J. Aviat. Med.* 9:92.

Ashley, F. W. Jr., and W. B. Kannel. 1974. Relation of weight change to changes in atherogenic traits; The Framingham study. *J. Chron. Dis.* 27:103.

Astrup, T., J. Rasmussen, and A. Amery. 1960. Fibrinolytic activity in cirrhosis of the liver. *Nature* 185:619.

Avtandilov, G. G. 1960. Klassifikatsiya i planimetricheskaya otsenka ateroskleroticheskikh porazhenii sosudov (Classification and planimetric assessment of atherosclerotic lesions in vessels). *Nauch. med. o-vo KB ASSR*, Nal'chik, 67 p.

Avtandilov, G. G. 1963. Osnovnye zakonomernosti vozrastnoi dinamiki razvitiya ateroskleroticheskikh porazhenii aorty i venechnykh arterii serdtsa (Fundamental rules of the age-related changes in the development of atherosclerotic lesions in the aorta and coronary arteries). *Arkh. Pat.*, 11:21.

Avtandilov, G. G. 1965. Sootnoshenie mezhdu osnovnymi vidami morfologicheskikh proyavlenii ateroskleroza v aorte i venechnykh arteriyakh serdtsa (The correlation between the principal types of morphologic changes in the aorta and coronary arteries). *Arkh. Pat.* 3:18.

Avtandilov, G. G. 1970. Dinamika ateroskleroticheskogo protsessa u cheloveka (Voprosy morfogeneza i patogeneza) (The dynamics of the atherosclerotic process in man—the problems of morphogenesis and pathogenesis). Meditsina, Moscow, p. 208.

Azerad, E., P. Kartun and J. Lubetzki. 1963. Diabete et atherosclerose. *Cocur Med. Intern.* 2:3.

Babushkina, L. G. 1966. Rol legkikh v zhirovom obmene i narushenii ego pri silikoze (The role of lungs in lipid metabolism and its disruption in silicosis). *Arkh. Pat.* 7:3.

Badmaeva, V. V. 1963. Ateroskleroz sonnykh arterii (Atherosclerosis of the carotid arteries), in *Gistokhimiya v patologicheskoii anatomii*. Moscow, p. 262.

Bahl, A. L. 1970. Preclinical diabetes mellitus in precocious myocardial infarction. *Brit. Heart J.* 32:701.

Bailey, N. 1962. Statisticheskie metody v biologii (Statistical methods in biology). Translated from English. *Izd. inostr. literat.* Moscow, p. 260.

Baizakova, S. S. 1967. Khronicheskie pnevmonii i ateroskleroz (Chronic lung disease and atherosclerosis), in *Sbornik rabot Kirgizsk. med. in-ta.* 43:145.

Balo, J. 1957. *Lungenkarzinom und Lungenadenom*. Budapest.

Bell, E. T. 1950. Incidence of gangrene of the extremities in nondiabetic and in diabetic persons. *Arch. Path.* 49:469.

Bell, E. T. 1952. A postmortem study of vascular disease in diabetes. *Arch. Path.* 53:444.

Benians, R. G. 1956. Tuberculous hypotension. *Brit. J. Tuber.* 50:152.

Berezhnitskii, M. N. 1962. Vliyanie gipoksii na plastichnost venechnykh arterii serdtsa pri kardiopul'monal'nom sindrome (The effect of hypoxia on the compliance of the coronary arteries in the cardiopulmonary syndrome). *Tezisy Nauchn. Konferentsii "Patologiya serdechnsosudistoi sistemy i gipoksiya."* Kiev, p. 21.

Bernick, S., P. Patek, B. Ershoff, and A. Wells. 1962. Effect of cholesterol feeding on the thyroid gland and vascular structures of the rabbit, guineapig, hamster, and rat. *Am. J. Path.* 41:661.

Bessmertnyi, B. S. 1967. Matematicheskaya statistika v klinicheskoi, profilakticheskoi i eksperimental'noi meditsine (Mathematical statistics in clinical, preventive, and experimental medicine). Meditsina, Moscow, 303 p.

Binet, L. 1935. Legkie kak zhelezistyi organ (The lungs as an endocrine organ), in *Problemy biologii i meditsiny*. Moscow, Leningrad, p. 419.

Bjurulf, P. 1964. Atherosclerosis in different parts of the arterial system. *Am. Heart J.* 68:41.

Blumenthal, H. T. 1968. The relation of microangiopathies to arteriosclerosis with special reference to diabetes. *Ann. N.Y. Acad. Sci.* 149:834.

Boas, E. P. 1952. Arteriosclerosis and diabetes. *J. Mt. Sinai Hosp.* 19:411.

Boiko, Yu. G. 1957. Gipertonicheskaya bolezn i sakharnyi diabet (Hypertension and diabetes mellitus). *Sov. med.* 5:61.

Boyd, G. S. 1961. The thyroid, iodothyroinines and atherosclerosis. *J. Atheroscler. Rev.* 1:26.

Braude, V. I. 1963. Atheroskleroz pri tuberkuleze legkikh (Atherosclerosis in pulmonary tuberculosis). *Sov. med.* 3:55.

Braude, V. I. 1966. Serdechno-sosudistye zabolevaniya v sochetanii s tuberkulezom legkikh (The cardiovascular diseases in combination with pulmonary tuberculosis). *Sov. med.* 12:104.

Brodsky, I., and L. H. Dennis. 1966. Evaluation of fibrinolysis in hepatic cirrhosis. *Am. J. Clin. Path.* 45:61.

Büchele, S. 1962. Über die Beziehung Zwischen Herzinfarkt und Diabetes mellitus unter besonderer Berucksichtingung des latenten Diabetes. *Schweiz. Med. Wschr.* 92:742.

Burstein, J., B. A. Lamberg, and E. Erämaa. 1960. Myocardial infarctions in thyrotoxicosis. *Acta Med. Scand.* 166:379.

Buschman, G., E. Fritze, and A. Marsch. 1958. Verlaufsbeobachtungen an 1500 Zuckerkranken. *Dtsch. Med. Wschr.* 30:1284.

Butkus, R. I. 1967. Funktsional'naya morfologiya vnutrisekretornogo apparata podzheludochnoi zhelezy pri ateroskleroze (Functional anatomy of the internal secretory apparatus of the pancreatic gland in atherosclerosis). Ph.D. thesis (abstract), Kaunas.

Buvailo, S. A. 1960. K metodike kolichestvennoi otsenki ateroskleroza (The method of quantitative assessment of atherosclerosis). *Arkh. Pat.* 5:83.

Camus, J. P. 1963. Les hypercalcémies. *Cahiers R.M.F.* 78:693.

Care, A. D., T. Duncan, and D. Webster. 1967. Thyrocalcitonin and its role in calcium homeostasis. *J. Endocr.* 37:155.

Chazov, E. I., A. M. Vikhert, and V. I. Metelitsa. 1972. Epidemiologiya ishemicheskoi bolezni serdtsa (Epidemiology of ischemic heart disease). *Kardiologiya* 8:134.

Chebotarev, D. F. 1959. Znachenie revmatizma v razvitii skleroticheskikh izmenenii aorty (The importance of rheumatic heart disease in the development of sclerotic changes in the aorta). *Vrach. delo.* 6:567.

Chernokanu, G. I. 1967. Funktsional'naya morfologiya shchitovidnoi zhelezy pri ateroskleroze (The functional morphology of the thyroid gland in atherosclerosis), in *Trudy 4-go Vsesoyuzn. S'ezda patologoanatomov*, Moscow, p. 78.

Chiari, H. 1928. Über Veranderungen in der Adventitia der Aorta und ihrer Hauptaste in Gefolge von Rheumatismus. *Beitr. Path. Anat.* 80:336.

Clawson, B. J., and E. T. Bell. 1949. Incidence of fatal coronary disease in nondiabetic persons. *Arch. Path.* 48:105.

Colleson, L., J. P. Grilliant, J. Mathieu, and J. Laurent. 1965. L'ostéose raréfiante dans les cirrhosis du foie. *Presse med.* 73:2571.

Cooper, G. R., C. B. Quinlan, V. S. Whiter, and G. I. Barrow. 1960. Atherogenesis and its relation to diabetes. *J. Med. Assn. Ga.* 49:99.

Corvilain, J. 1967. La thyrocalcitonine. *Acta Clin. Belg.* 22:308.

Creed, D. L., W. F. Baird, and E. R. Fischer. 1955. The severity of aortic arteriosclerosis in certain diseases; a necropsy study. *Am. J. Med. Sci.* 230:385.

Czerkawski, J. W. 1963. Diabetes and vascular degeneration, in *International review of connective tissue research* (D. A. Hall, ed.). New York, p. 307.

Damir, A. M., and G. E. Sarankin. 1963. Koronarnoe krovoobrashchenie u bol'nykh pnevmosklerozom u pozhilykh (The coronary circulation in elderly patients with pneumosclerosis). *Ter. Arkh.* 2:16.

Danilova, R. A., N. A. Talikov, V. P. Tikhonov, T. G. Danilova, T. M. Mirazimov, I. Fakhtullaev, and L. G. Kirillova. 1967. K voprosu o morfologii zhelez vnutrennei sekretsii pri ateroskleroze (The morphology of the endocrine glands in atherosclerosis), in *Trudy 4-go Vsesoyuzn. S'ezda patologoanatomov*. Moscow, p. 56.

Davidenkova, E. F. 1970. Genetika sakharnogo diabeta (Etiology of diabetes mellitus). *Vest. AMN SSSR* 1:78.

Davis, D., and N. J. Klainer. 1940. Studies in hypertensive heart disease. *Am. Heart J.* 19:185.

Davydovskii, I. V. 1958. *Patologicheskaya anatomiya i patogenez boleznei cheloveka* (*Pathological anatomy and the pathogenesis of human diseases*), vol. II. Medgiz, 692 p.

Davydovskii, I. V. 1967. Ateroskleroz kak problema vozrasta (Atherosclerosis as an aging problem), in *Trudy 4-go Vsesoyuzn. S'ezda patologoanatomov*. Moscow, p. 10.

Della Salda, C. 1966. Miocardiopatic e infarto nel diabetico. *Cardiol. Prat.* (Firenze) 17:53.

Deming, Q. B. 1966. Experimental atherosclerosis and hypertension, in *Antihypertensive therapy, Principles and Practice* (F. Gross, ed.). Springer Verlag, Berlin, p. 11.

Dixon, K. 1961. Deposition of globular lipid in arterial cells in relation to anoxia. *Am. J. Path.* 39:65.

Doerr, W. 1963. *Perfusiontheorie der Arteriosklerosis*. Stuttgart.

Duff, G. L., and T. P. Pyne. 1950. The effects of alloxan diabetes on experimental cholesterol atherosclerosis in the rabbit. *J. Exp. Med.* 92:299.

Dungal, N., and T. Benedictsson. 1958. Gastric cancer and atherosclerosis. *Lancet* 1:931.

Eakins, D. 1965. Atherosclerosis and malignant disease. *Brit. J. Cancer*, 19:9.

Egorov, B. A. 1936. *Revmatizm serdtsa i sosudov* (*Rheumatic disease of the heart and vessels*). Biomedgiz, Moscow, 215 p.

Egorova, E. M., and R. A. Mezentsev. 1962. Patogeneticheskaya svyaz sakharnogo diabeta i ateroskleroza (The pathogenetic relationship between diabetes mellitus and atherosclerosis). *Ter. Arkh.* 8:67.

Eilerson, P., and M. Faber. 1960. The human aorta. 6. The regression of atherosclerosis in pulmonary tuberculosis. *Arch. Path.* 70:103.

Eliasch, H., O. Edhag, A. Grepe, and G. Biorck. 1967. Contribution of the coronary arteriogram to diagnosis of coronary atherosclerosis in coronary heart disease. *Am. J. Cardiol.* 19:502.

Elkeles, A. 1953. Peptic ulcer in the aged and gastric carcinoma and their relationship to atherosclerosis: roentgenological study. *Am. J. Roentgenol.* 70:787.

Elkeles, A. 1963. Calcified atherosclerosis and cancer of low malignancy. *Brit. J. Cancer*, 17:572.

Evans, P. H. 1965. Relation of longstanding blood pressure level to atherosclerosis. *Lancet* 1:516.

Evdokimov, N. M. 1968. Sostoyanie svertyvayushchei i antisvertyvayushchei sistem krovi pri grippe i nekotorykh legochnykh zabolevaniyakh (The coagulation and anticoagulation process in influenza and in some lung diseases). Abstract of Ph.D. thesis, Leningrad.

Evnina, I. I., E. I. Ivashkevich, V. S. Sergeevskii, and E. Ya. Skribnik. 1967. O funktsional'nom sostoyanii kory nadpochechnikov pri mitral'nom poroke serdtsa (The activity of the adrenal cortex in mitral valve disease). *Klin. med.* 3:98.

Faber, M., and F. Lund. 1951. The human aorta, 4. The aorta in diabetes mellitus. *Arch. Path.* 52:239.

Fanconi, G. 1960. Calcium and phosphorus metabolism. *S. Afr. Med. J.* 34:769.

Farquhar, W., R. I. Hirsch, and Ahrens, Jr. 1960. Evidence that atheromatous fatty acids are in flux. *J. Clin. Invest.* 39:984.

Feldman, M., and M. Feldman, Jr. 1954. The association of coronary occlusion and infarction in diabetes mellitus. A necropsy study. *Am. J. Med. Sci.* 228:53.

Fischer, E. R. 1961. The effect of hypertension on cholesterol atherosclerosis in diabetic rabbits. *Lab. Invest.* 10:361.

Fischer, E. R. 1964. Thyroidal influence in experimental cholesterol atherosclerosis. *Am. J. Path.* 45:21.

Fischer, E. R. 1965. Cholesterol atherosclerosis in rabbits with cirrhosis. *Am. J. Path.* 46:577.

Fishberg, A. M. 1944. *Hypertension and nephritis.* Lea and Febiger, Philadelphia.

Fletcher, A. P., O. Biderman, Don Moore, N. Alkjaersik, and S. Sherry. 1964. Abnormal plasminogen plasmin system activity (fibrinolysis) in patients with hepatic cirrhosis. *J. Clin. Invest.* 43:681.

Fletcher, K., and N. B. Myant. 1962. Effects of thyroxine on the synthesis of lipids in rat liver. *Endocrinology* 71:870.

Fomenko, L. P., and T. N. Tirkina. 1971. Kharakter i chastota gipertonii u bol'nykh sakharnym diabetom (The nature and prevalence of hypertension in patients with diabetes mellitus). *Ter. Arkh.* 7:17.

Fotopoulous, I. P., A. R. Crampton, and H. C. Burkhead. 1962. Calcification of the abdominal aorta as an aid in the diagnosis of gastric carcinoma vs. benign ulcer. *Radiology* 79:637.

Fox, S. M., and O. Paul. 1969. Physical activity and coronary heart disease. *Am. J. Cardiol.* 23:298.

Frank, C. W., and A. Einstein. 1968. The course of coronary heart disease: factors relating to prognosis. *Bull. N.Y. Acad. Med.* 44:900.

Freis, E. D. 1969. Hypertension and atherosclerosis. *Am. J. Med.* 46:735.

Freudenberg, K. 1958. Arteriosclerose und Krebs. *Z. Krebsforschr.* 62:527.

Fridlyand, I. B. 1927. Rol shchitovidnoi zhelezy v patogeneze ateroskleroza (The role of the thyroid gland in the pathogenesis of atherosclerosis). *Klin. Med.* 24:1300.

Fuks, B. B., and F. I. Leites. 1967. Ob otnoshenii adaptivnogo sisteza belkov-fermentov k patogenezu ateroskleroza (The relationship of adaptation of proteolytic enzymes to the pathogenesis of atherosclerosis), in *Trudy 4-go Vsesoyuzn. S''ezda patologoanatomov*, Moscow, p. 38.

Funk, H. U. 1965. Veränderungen an Kleinen Extremitätengefassen von Diabetikern. *Schweitz. Med. Wschr.* 95:487.

Gamiyants, S. A. 1964. K voprosy o sochetanii aterosklerotichеskogo porazheniya sosudov so zlokachestvennymi novoobrazovaniyami (The problem of combinations of atherosclerotic lesions with malignant neoplasms), in *Materialy I-i Konferentsii patologoanatomov Uzbeksk.* SSR. Tashkent, p. 43.

Gandzha, I. M. 1961. *Serdechno-sosudistaya sistema pri bolezni pecheni i zhelchnykh putei* (The cardiovascular system in diseases of the liver and bile ducts). Gosmedizdat Uk. SSR, Kiev, 157 p.

Ganelina, I. E., and I. N. Komarova. 1963. Shchitovidnaya zheleza, obmen lipidov i ateroskleroz (The thyroid gland, lipid metabolism, and atherosclerosis). *Probl. endokrinol.* 1:113.

Genes, S. G. 1963. *Sakharnyi diabet* (*Diabetes mellitus*). Medgiz, Moscow, 378 p.

Gerasimchuk, R. D. 1966. Arterial'noe davlenie u bol'nykh tuberkulezom legkikh (Blood pressure of patients with pulmonary tuberculosis). *Sov. Med.* 7:48.

Giertsen, J. C. 1966. Atherosclerosis in an autopsy series. 8. Relation of malignant disease to atherosclerosis. *Acta Path. Microbiol. Scand.* 66:341.

Giertsen, J. C. 1966. Atherosclerosis in an autopsy series. 9. The relation of atherosclerosis of the heart to atherosclerosis. *Acta Path. Microbiol. Scand.* 66:351.

Giertsen, J. C. 1966. Atherosclerosis in an autopsy series. 10. Relation of nutritional state to atherosclerosis. 11. General summary and conclusion. *Acta Path. Microbiol. Scand.* 67:305.

Gimbashidze, N. B. 1967. Rol'gipofizarno-tireoidnoi sistemy v mekhanizme deistviya polovykh gormonov pri eksperimental'nom ateroskleroze koronarnykh arterii (The role of the hypophyseal-thyroid system in the mechanism of action of sex hormones in experimental coronary atherosclerosis, in *Ateroskleroz i koronarnaya nedostatochnost*. Tbilisi, p. 227.

Gitters, R. F., and G. L. Irvin. 1966. Role of thyroxine and thyrocalcitonin in the response to hypercalcemia in rats. *Endocrinology* 79:1033.

Glagov, S. 1965. Hemodynamic factors in the localization of atherosclerosis. *Acta Cardiol.* (Brux.), 20 (11):311.

Glazunov, I. S. 1961. Rasprostranenie infarkta miokarda sredi naseleniya nekotorykh gorodov SSSR v svyazi s urovnem kholesterina krovi i pitaniem (Distribution of myocardial infarction in the population of several cities of the USSR and its relation to the level of serum cholesterol and diet). Abstract of Ph.D. thesis, Moscow.

Golden, J. B., and E. I. Sevringhaus. 1938. Inactivation of estrogenic hormone of the ovary by the liver. *Proc. Soc. Exp. Biol.* (N.Y.) 39:361.

Goldschmidt, R. 1934. Über den Antagonismus Zwischen dem Morbus Basedowii und der Atherosclerosis. Diss. Berlin.

Goodman, J. I., S. Wasserman, L. J. Markus, and L. Frankel. 1950. A study of atherosclerosis in a group of diabetic patients. *Am. J. Med. Sci.* 220:30.

Goryachkina, L. N. 1970. Osobennosti razvitiya ateroskleroza u bol'nykh khronicheskoi pnevmoniei (The characteristics of the development of atherosclerosis in patients with COPD). Abstract of Ph.D. thesis, Irkutsk.

Grigor'eva, V. A. 1967. Svertyvayushchaya i protivosvertyvayushchaya sistema krovi u bol'nykh revmaticheskimi porokami serdtsa i ikh izmeneniya pri lechenii antikoagulyantami (The coagulation and anticoagulation system in patients with rheumatic heart disease and their treatment with anticoagulants). *Ter. Arkh.* 1:75.

Gritting, G., and H. A. Salvesen. 1957. Thyrotoxicosis and myocardial infarction. *Acta Med. Scand.* 157:169.

Grollman, A. 1962. The role of cholesterol in the body. *Med. Ann. D.C.* 31:129.

Gross, H., and B. S. Oppenheimer. 1936. The significance of rheumatic fever in the etiology of coronary artery disease and thrombosis. *Am. Heart J.* 11:648.

Grosse, H. 1960. Krebssyntropien. Wahiverwandtschaften und Lokalisations gesetze des Krebses. Jena.

Grosse, H. 1964. Über die Syntropie von Leberzirrhose und Myokardinfarkt. *Z. Kreisl. Forschr.* 53:677.

Gruzina, E. A., G. F. Boiko, R. A. Tregubenko, and V. I. Pantyukhin. 1974. O faktorakh sposobstvuyshchikh razvitiyu ateroskleroza pri sakharnom diabete (The factors predisposing to the development of atherosclerosis in diabetes mellitus). *Vrach. delo.* 2:46.

Gubler, E. V., and A. A. Genkin, 1973. *Primenenie neparametricheskikh kriteriev statistiki v medikobiologicheskikh issledovaniyakh* (*Application of non-parametric criteria of statistics in medicobiological studies*). Meditsina, Leningrad, 141 p.

Gurova, A. M., and A. A. Abramova. 1945. Kliniko-anatomicheskie dannye o koronarnom ateroskleroze u bol'nykh tireotoksikozom (The clinico-anatomical data on coronary atherosclerosis in patients with thyrotoxicosis). *Klin. Med.* 3:28.

Haber, J., and E. Marton. 1963. Arteriosclerosis es tuberkulozis. *Tuberkulozis* 16:25.

Haimovici, H. 1961. Peripheral arterial disease in diabetes. *N.Y. St. J. Med.* 61:2988.

Hall, E. M., A. Y. Otsen, and F. E. Davis. 1953. Portal cirrhosis. Clinical and pathologic review of 782 cases from 16,600 necropsies. *Am. J. Path.* 29:993.

Hamburger, J., G. Richet, J. Grosnier, and J. L. Funck-Brentano. 1965. *L'insuffisance renale*. Translated from French. Meditsina, Moscow.

Harrison, C. V., and P. Wood. 1949. Hypertensive and ischemic heart diseases: a comparative clinical and pathological study. *Brit. Heart J.* 11:205.

Hart, J. F., and J. R. Lisa. 1944. Diabetes mellitus and arteriosclerosis—the effect of duration and severity on arterial changes. *N.Y. St. J. Med.* 44:2479.

Hass, G. M., D. E. Hensson, R. A. Scott, E. C. McClain, and A. Hemmens. 1969. Influence of cirrhosis on production of athero-arteriosclerosis and thromboarteritis. Vitamin D and dietary cholesterol. *Am. J. Path.* 57:405.

Hempel, K. I. 1957. Zur Frage besonderer Typen der Arteriosklerosa. *Z. Ges. Inn. Med.* 12:740.

Henshen, P. 1961. Sootnoshenii ateroskleroza s vozrastom, polom, tuberkulezom, i opukholyami (The correlation of atherosclerosis with age, sex, tuberculosis, and tumors). *Trudy voen-med akad. im S.M. Kirova* 131:33.

Hirst, A. E., G. G. Hadley, and I. Gore. 1965. The effect of chronic alcoholism and cirrhosis of the liver on atherosclerosis. *Am. J. Med. Sci.* 249:143.

Hodler, J. 1963. Diabetes und Gefasserkrankungen. *Schweiz. Med. Wschr.* 93:526.

Holle, G. 1943. Über Lipoidose, Atheromathose und Sklerose der Aorta und deren Beziehung zur Endokarditis. *Virch. Arch. Path. Anat.* 310:160.

Holle, G., and B. Nierade. 1963. Über Beziehungen Zwischen Aortensklerose und Mesaortitis Chronica Rheumatica. *Zbl. Allg. Path.* 105:16.

Holman, R. L. 1960. An index for the evaluation of atherosclerotic lesions in the abdominal aorta. *Circulation* 22:1137.

Holman, R. L., H. C. MacGill, J. P. Strong, and J. C. Geer. 1958. Techniques for studying atherosclerotic lesions. *Lab. Invest.* 7:42.

Horn, V. 1959. Histologickezmen plicnich a jinych organovych arterii pri revmatickem onemocheni srdu. *Cas. Lek. Ces.* 3:76.

Howell, W. L., and W. C. Manion. 1960. The low incidence of myocardial infarction in patients with cirrhosis of the liver. *Am. Heart J.* 60:341.

Il'inskii, B. V. 1960. *Ateroskleroz* (*Atherosclerosis*). Medgiz, Leningrad, 333 p.

Il'inskii, B. V., and B. S. Nalimov. 1966. Chastota ateroskleroza pri tuberkuleže (The prevalence of atherosclerosis in tuberculosis), in *Trudy Leningradsk. nauch. o-va patologoanatomov*, Leningrad, p. 25.

Il'inskii, B. V., and G. N. Vereshchagina. 1967. O roli pecheni v razvitii ateroskleroza (The role of the liver in the development of atherosclerosis). *Kardiologiya* 4:25.

Il'yasov, L. Kh. 1966. Funktsional'noe sostoyanie svertyvayushchei i protivo-svertyvayushchei sistem krovi pri khronicheskikh nespetsificheskikh zabolevaniyakh legkikh (The condition of the coagulation and anticoagulation processes in chronic nonspecific diseases of the lungs). Abstract of Ph.D. thesis, Baku.

Jonas, V., and L. Kozak. 1963. Izuchenie izmenenii sosudov u diabetikov (The study of vascular changes in diabetics). *Czechoslovak. Med. Obzor* 3:173.

Jonas, V., and L. Kozak. 1966. Sakharnyi diabet i ateroskleroz. O serdechnom infarkte u diabetikov (Diabetes mellitus and atherosclerosis. Myocardial infarction in diabetics). *Kardiologiya* 3:16.

Joslin, E. P. 1961. Diabetes in the future. *Diabetes* 10:148.

Joslin, E. P., H. F. Root, P. White, and A. Marble. 1959. *The treatment of diabetes mellitus.* Philadelphia.

Jowett, M. 1931. The phosphatide and cholesterol contents of normal and malignant human tissues. *Biochem. J.* 25:1991.

Juhl, S. 1955. Cancer and atherosclerosis. Negative correlation. *Acta Path. Microbiol. Scand.* 37:166.

Juhl, S. 1957. Cancer and atherosclerosis. 2. Applicability of postmortem statistics in the study of the negative correlation. *Acta Path. Microbiol. Scand.* 41:99.

Kadas, I. 1961. Beitrage Verhaltnis von Krebs und Arteriosklerose. *Zbl. Allg. Path.* 102:450.

Kagan, A., and K. Uemura. 1962. Grading atherosclerosis in the aorta and coronary arteries obtained at autopsy. *Bull. WHO* 27:667.

Kannel, N. B., W. P. Castelli, and P. M. McNamara. 1968. Epidemiology of acute myocardial infarction. *Medicine Today* 2:56.

Karsner, H. T., and F. Baylers. 1934. The coronary arteries in rheumatic fever. *Am. Heart J.* 9:557.

Kasatkina, I. V. 1969. Rol' osnovnogo veshchestva arterii v patogeneze ateroskleroza (The role of the principal metabolic factors in the pathogenesis of atherosclerosis). Abstract of D.Sc. thesis, Moscow.

Katsuki, S., T. Omae, and J. Hirota. 1964. Epidemiological and clinicopathological studies of cerebrovascular disease. *Kyushu J. Med. Sci.* 15:127.

Kazykhanov, N. S. 1967. Ateroskleroz u bol'nykh tuberkulezom legkikh (Atherosclerosis in patients with pulmonary tuberculosis). *Kardiologiya* 10:137.

Kerner, Yu. M. 1930. Formy i sushchnost' lipoidnoi infil'tratsii aorty v svyazi s kolichestovom i lokalizatsiei legochnogo tuberkuleza (The nature of lipid deposition in the aorta depending on the degree and localization of pulmonary tuberculosis). *Vopr. Tub.* 11–12:12.

Kettler, L. H. 1970. (Hrg.) *Lehrbuch der speziellen Pathologie*. Jena.

Khasanov, A. P. 1959. Morfologicheskaya kharakteristika tuberkuloza i ego oslozhnenii u vzroslykh po sektsionnym dannym Leningrada 1953–1967 gg (Morphological characteristics of tuberculosis and its complications in adults in selected material from Leningrad, 1953 through 1967). *Probl. Tub.* 8:75.

Kipshidze, N. N. 1959. Vliyanie kislorodnogo golodaniya na razvitie eksperimental'nogo ateroskleroza koronarnykh arterii (The effect of oxygen deficiency on the development of experimental coronary atherosclerosis). *Byull. Eksper. Biol.* 4:54.

Klemashev, I. S. 1964. O nekotorykh osobennostyakh ateroskleroza arterii nizhnikh konechnostei pri sakharnom diabete po dannym arteriografii (Some angiographic features of atherosclerosis in the arteries of the lower extremities in diabetes mellitus). *Probl. Endokrinol.* 5:17.

Klinge, E. 1933. Der Rheumatismus. *Egebn. Allg. Path. Anat.* 27:1.

Klotz, O. 1926. Arteriosclerosis. *Canad. Med. Ass. J.* 16:11.

Kochetov, A. M., I. I. Bykov, I. M. Kumonok, N. I. Kaz, and E. K. Khmel'nitskii. 1970. O rasprostranennosti ateroskleroza aorty i venechnykh arterii serdtsa pri rake organov pishchevareniya (The extent of atherosclerosis in the aorta and coronary arteries in carcinoma of the digestive organs). *Krovoobrashchenie* (Yerevan) 5:28.

Kogan, B. B., B. S. Khodzhamirova, L. A. Gulina, and V. S. Zhdanov. 1960. Diabeticheskii glomeruloskleroz (Diabetic glomerulosclerosis). *Ter. Arkh.* 2:16.

Kogan, M. B. 1936. Glikemicheskie reaktsii i ikh znachenie v simptomatologii i klinike grudnoi zhaby (Glycemic reactions and their significance in angina pectoris). *Klin. Med.* 6:777.

Kogan-Yasnyi, V. M. 1957. *Sakharnaya bolezn'* (*Diabetes mellitus*). Medgiz, Moscow, p. 302.

Kolomoiskaya, M. B. 1964. O vozmozhnosti sochetaniya khronicheskikh nespetsificheskikh zabolevanii legkikh s aterosklerozom (Features of the combination of chronic nonspecific diseases of the lungs with atherosclerosis). *Ter. Arkh.* 2:100.

Kononyachenko, V. A. 1971. *Gipertonicheskaya bolezn' i simptomaticheskie gipertonii* (*Hypertension and secondary hypertension*). Medgiz, Moscow.

Kraevskii, N. A. 1937. Anatomoklinicheskii analiz revmaticheskogo kardita (The clinico-anatomical analysis of rheumatic carditis). *Arkh. Pat.* 1:5.

Kremnev, T. I. 1951. In: *Voprosy kliniki i patologii serdechnososudistoi sistemy* (*The clinical features and pathology of the cardiovascular system*). Kursk. p. 30.

Kulachkovskii, Yu. V. 1967. Kora nadpochechnikov i ee gormony pri khronicheskom logochnom serdtse bol'nykh tuberkulezom legkikh (The adrenal cortex and its hormones in patients with chronic cor pulmonale with pulmonary tuberculosis). *Vrach. delo* 10:68.

Kumonok, I. M. 1967. Chastota i rasprostranennost ateroskleroza pri pervichnom rake legkikh (The prevalence and distribution of atherosclerosis in primary carcinoma of the lungs). *Vrach. delo* 3:57.

Kushelevskii, B. P., and A. M. Gurova. 1966. Infarkt miokarda u bol'nykh tireotoksikozom (Myocardial infarction in patients with thyrotoxicosis). *Kardiologiya* 1:65.

Kushnir, V. E., and Yu. S. Kozachuk. 1966. O rasslaivayushchei anevrizme aorty pri revmatizme (Dissecting aneurysm of the aorta in rheumatic disease). *Vopr. revmat.* 4:70.

Kyeldsen, J., Wanstrup, and P. Astrup. 1968. Enhancing influence of arterial hypoxia on the development of atherosclerosis in cholesterol-fed rabbits. *J. Atheroscler. Res.* 8:835.

Lashchetko, E. L. 1964. O soputstvuyushchikh zabolevaniyakh pri tuberkuleze legkikh (Associated diseases in pulmonary tuberculosis), in *Khimiya i meditsina*, Riga, p. 52.

Lauchevichus, L. Z., Sh. A. Suderaite, and D. V. Triponeze. 1973. O vzaimosvyazi sakharnogo diabeta i ateroskleroza (The interrelationship of diabetes mellitus and atherosclerosis). *Klin. Med.* 2:115.

Le Compte, Ph. M. 1945. Vascular lesions in diabetes mellitus. *J. Chron. Dis.* 2:178.

Leites, F. I. 1967. *Gistokhimiya lipoliticheskikh fermentov v norme i pri patologii lipoidnogo obmena* (*Histochemistry of lipolytic enzymes in normal and in pathological lipid metabolism*). Meditsina, Moscow, 248 p.

Leites, S. M. 1966. *Patofiziologiya kholesterinovogo obmena* (Pathophysiology of cholesterol metabolism), Tsentr. in-t usover. vrachei, Moscow, 44 p.

Leites, Sh. M. 1932. Chastota ateroskleroza u rakovykh bol'nykh po sektsionnym dannym (The prevalence of atherosclerosis in cancer patients as indicated by autopsy). *Vestn. rentgenol.* 10:229.

Leupold, F., and H. D. Kenk. 1965. Die Lipoidzusammensetzung von normalen und pathologische Lebern des Menschen. *Dtsch. Arch. Klin. Med.* 210:238.

Liberman, I. S. 1965. O nekotorykh kliniko-geneticheskikh formakh sakharnogo diabeta (Some forms of clinicogenetical diabetes mellitus). *Vestn. AMN SSSR* 3:37.

Libiyainen, T. P. 1963. Rasslaivayushchaya s razryvom anevrizma bryushnoi aorty na pochve revmaticheskogo aortita (Rupture of a dissecting aneurysm of the abdominal aorta in rheumatic aortitis), in *Trudy Ryazansk. med. in-ta.* 14:96.

Liebow, I. M., and H. K. Hellerstein. 1949. Cardiac complications of diabetes mellitus. *Am. J. Med.* 7:660.

Liebow, I. M., H. K. Hellerstein, and M. Miller. 1955. Arteriosclerotic heart disease in diabetes mellitus. *Am. J. Med.* 18:438.

Lifshits, A. M., Yu. I. Zinenko, G. G. Avtandilov, and O. V. Ponomarenko. 1966. Vizual'nyi i planimetricheskii metody otsenki stepeni ateroskleroza (Visual and planimetric methods for assessment of the degree of atherosclerosis). *Arkh. Pat.* 9:72.

Labova, I. V. 1969. O chastote i vyrazhennosti ateroskleroza arterii bol'shogo kruga krovoobrashcheniya u bol'nykh khronicheskoi pnevmoniei (The prevalence and degree of atherosclerosis of the systemic arteries in patients with chronic lung disease). *Ter. Arkh.* 3:68.

Loginov, A. S., and I. I. Yutanova. 1967. K voprosu ob ateroskleroze pri tsirrozakh pecheni (Atherosclerosis in cirrhosis of the liver). *Kardiologiya* 4:29.

Lomazova, Kh. D. 1963. Pechen' i svertyvanie krovi (The liver and blood coagulation). *Uspekhi sovr. biol.* 3:418.

Loyke, H. F. 1955. The relationship of cirrhosis of the liver to hypertension: a study of 504 cases of cirrhosis of the liver. *Am. J. Med. Sci.* 230:627.

Lubetzki, J. 1973. Diabète et athérosclérose. *Concour Med. Intern.* 12:183.

Lukash, N. V., and R. A. Kaganovich. 1965. Vliyanie zabolevanii pecheni i zhelchnykh putei na razvitie ateroskleroza (The effect of liver and bile ducts diseases on the development of atherosclerosis). *Arkh. Pat.* 12:63.

Lundback, K., and V. P. Peterson. 1953. Lipid composition of diabetic and nondiabetic coronary arteries. *Acta Med. Scand.* 144:354.

Lunseth, J. H., E. G. Olmstead, and F. Abboud. 1958. A study of heart disease in one hundred eight hospitalized patients dying with portal cirrhosis. *Arch. Intern. Med.* 102:405.

MacDonald, R. A., and G. K. Mallory. 1958. The natural history of postnecrotic cirrhosis. *Am. J. Med.* 24:334.

Mad'yar, I. 1961. Diabet i arterioskleroz (Diabetes and atherosclerosis). *Vestn. AMN SSSR* 3:3.

Maher, J., and L. Schreier. 1957. Pathogenesis of atherosclerosis in youth. *Circulation* 16:492.

Maksudov, B. S. 1960. Funktsional'noe sostoyanie shchitovidnoi zhelezy u krolikov pri dlitel'noi giperkholesterinemii i vyrazhennom ateroskleroze (The functional status of the thyroid gland of rabbits in prolonged hypercholesterolemia and pronounced atherosclerosis). *Probl. Endokrinol.* 1:38.

Matova, E. E. 1972. Ateroskleroz aorty i venechnykh arterii serdtsa pri arterial'nykh gipertoniyakh razlichnoi etiologii (Atherosclerosis of the aorta and coronary arteries in arterial hypertension of varying etiology). Abstract of D.Sc. thesis, Moscow.

Medes, G. A., T. Weinhouse, and S. Weinhouse. 1953. Metabolism of neoplastic tissue. IV. A study of lipid synthesis in neoplastic tissue slices *in vitro*. *Cancer Res.* 13:27.

Medvedeva, N. B. 1955. Normal'naya i patologicheskaya fiziologiya zhirovogo i lipoidnogo obmena (Normal and pathological physiology of the fat and lipoid metabolism). Izd. AN USSR, Kiev, 365 p.

Merriggi, A. 1960. Sui rapporti fra aterosclerosi aortica e cancro polmonare. *Riv. Anat. Pat.* 17:667.

Metelitsa, V. I. 1964. Vliyanie toksicheskogo porazheniya pecheni na razvitie eksperimental'nogo kholesterinovogo ateroskleroza u krolikov (The effect of toxic lesions of the liver on the development of experimental cholesterol atherosclerosis in rabbits). Abstract of Ph.D. thesis, Moscow.

Mezinova, N. N., and O. G. Khan. 1972. Ekskretsiya s mochoi estrogenov u bol'nykh rakom endometriya klimaktericheskogo i menopauzal'nogo vozrastnykh periodov (Urinary excretion of estrogens in patients of climacteric and menopausal age with endometrial carcinoma). *Akush. gin.* 10:21.

Mikhailenko, T. I. 1959. Prichiny smerti bol'nykh sakharnym diabetom (The causes of death of patients with diabetes mellitus), in *Sovremennye voprosy fiziologii i patologii endokrinnykh zhelez*. Khar'kov, p. 100.

Mikhailov, G. 1966. *Mezhdunarodnyi simpozium po gistologii*. Sofia.

Mikhnev, A. I., V. P. Bezuglyi, and N. V. Osabchaya. 1961. Rol' gipoksii v razvitii ateroskleroza (Role of hypoxia in the development of atherosclerosis). *Vrach. delo* 7:8.

Mikunis, R. I. 1963. O sostoyanii lipoidnogo obmena v raznykh formakh revmaticheskogo protsessa (Lipid metabolism in various types of rheumatism). *Ter. Arkh.* 10:131.

Mironov, I. I. 1963. Morfologicheskie izmeneniya v sisteme gipofiz—kora nadpochechnikov

pri revmatizme (Morphological changes in the hypophyseal-adrenal system in rheumatism), in *Trudy Ryazansk. Med. in-ta.*, Ryazan, vol. 14, p. 74.
Mitchell, J. R. A. 1971. Hypertension and arterial disease. *Brit. Heart J.* 33(Suppl.):122.
Mitchell, J. R. A., and C. J. Schwartz. 1965. *Arterial disease.* Oxford.
Mitchell, J. R. A., C. J. Schwartz, and A. Zinger. 1964. Relationship between aortic plaques and age, sex, and blood pressure. *Brit. Med. J.* 1:205.
Mitin, K. S. 1966. *Gistokhimiya soedinitel'noi tkani sosudov pri revmatizme* (*Histochemistry of the connective tissue of the vessels in rheumatic disease.* Meditsina, Moscow, 210 p.
Mohnike, G. 1957. Zur diabetischen Blutgefasskrankheit. *Dtsch. Med. Wschr.* 22:1904.
Moiseenko, V. M. 1970. Lipidnyi obmen u bol'nykh khronicheskimi vospalitel'nymi bronkholegochnymi zabolevaniyami i rakom legkikh (Fat metabolism in patients with chronic lung diseases and pulmonary carcinoma). Ph.D. thesis. Barnaul.
Montenegro, M. R., and L. A. Solberg. 1968. Obesity, body weight, body length, and atherosclerosis. *Lab. Invest.* 13:594.
Morehead, R. P. 1965. *Human pathology.* McGraw-Hill, New York.
Moschkowitz, E. 1951. The relation of hyperplastic arteriosclerosis to diabetes mellitus. *Ann. Intern. Med.* 34:1137.
Moses, C. 1963. *Atherosclerosis. Mechanisms as a guide to prevention.* Lea & Febiger, Philadelphia.
Mosinger, B., J. Pechar, and N. Segova. 1964. Some characteristics of the lipolytic activity of the rat and the human lung. *Physiol. Bohemoslov.* 13:300.
Moskovich, E. G. 1958. Sakharnyi diabet i ateroskleroz (Diabetes mellitus and atherosclerosis). *Klin. Med.* 10:76.
Möttönen, M. 1969. Myocardial infarction and coronary atherosclerosis in Finland. *Acta Path. Microbiol. Scand.* 205(Suppl.):84.
Mutina, E. S. 1968. Lipidy syvorotki pri ateroskleroze v sochetanii s gipertonicheskoi bolezn'yu i pri khronicheskikh netuberkuleznykh zabolevaniyakh legkikh (Serum lipids in atherosclerosis in combination with hypertension and chronic non-tuberculous diseases of the lungs). *Kardiologiya* 2:62.
Myant, B. 1964. The thyroid and lipid metabolism, in *Lipid Pharmacology* (G. E. Cronheim, ed.). New York, 299.
Myasnikov, A. L. 1956. *Bolezni pecheni i zhelchnykh putei* (*Diseases of the liver and bile ducts*). Medgiz, Moscow, 290 p.
Myasnikov, A. L. 1960. *Ateroskleroz* (*Atherosclerosis*). Medgiz, Moscow, 444 p.
Myasnikov, A. L. 1965. *Gipertonicheskaya bolezn' i ateroskleroz* (*Hypertension and atherosclerosis*). Meditsina, Moscow, 615 p.
Myasnikov, L. A. 1969. *Nervno-endokrinnye faktory pri ateroskleroze* (*Neuro-endocrine factors in atherosclerosis*). Meditsina, Moscow, 192 p.
Myasnikov, L. A., and I. C. Klemashev. 1965. Ateroskleroz pri sakharnom diabete (Atherosclerosis in diabetes mellitus). *Sov. Med.* 4:57.
Myasnikov, L. A., and V. I. Pyatenko. 1962. Tiretoksikoz i ateroskleroz (Thyrotoxicosis and atherosclerosis). *Ter. Arkh.* 4:57.
Myasnikov, L. A., L. V. Kasatkina, and E. N. Nikolaeva. 1971. K mekhanizmu usilivayushchego vliyaniya arterial'noi gipertonii na ateroskleroz (The mechanism of the intensifying effect of arterial hypertension on atherosclerosis). *Kardiologiya* 3:31.
Myasnikov, L. A., V. F. Zaitsev, and V. J. Metelitsa. 1967. Nekotorye problemy v izuchenii ateroskleroza (Some problems in the study of atherosclerosis), in *Ateroskleroz i koronarnaya nedostatochnost'*. Tbilisi, p. 15.
Naide, M. 1945. Diabetes mellitus as observed in 100 cases for 10 or more years; peripheral vascular findings in 84 of these cases. *Am. J. Med. Sci.* 209:23.

Nathanson, M. H. 1932. Coronary disease in 100 autopsied diabetics. *Am. J. Med. Sci.* 183:495.

Naunyn, B. 1906. *Der Diabetes mellitus.* Wien.

Nepryakhin, G. G. 1966. Ateroskleroz pri revmatizme (Atherosclerosis in rheumatic disease). *Arkh. Pat.* 12:3.

Nepryakhin, G. G., and A. A. Akhmetzyanov. 1966. Ateroskleroz pri revmatizme i tuberkuleze (Atherosclerosis in rheumatic disease and tuberculosis). *Kazansk. med. zh.* 5:8.

Nielsen, B. L., and S. V. Kersing. 1965. Hepatic cirrhosis and atherosclerotic heart disease. *Geriatrics* 20:344.

Nonkin, P. M., M. M. Dick, and G. L. Bam. 1964. Myocardial infarction in respiratory insufficiency. *Arch. Intern. Med.* 113:42.

Novikov, S. A., V. V. Sitnik, and A. A. Nikolaev. 1967. Zabolevaemost infarktom miokarda v Irkutske (Myocardial infarction in Irkutsk), in *Voprosy serdechnososudistoi patologii.* Irkutsk, p. 60.

Obraztsova, M. S., P. S. Semenova, and V. T. Rogova. 1965. Revmatizm v pozhilom vozraste (Rheumatic diseases in elderly subjects), in *Problemy geriatrii v klinike vnutrennikh boleznei.* Kiev, p. 244.

Ochkur, P. P., F. I. Gzulya, A. I. Zikeeva, G. N. Kiikbaeva, D. S. Lobanov, Yu. F. Lomakin, and B. I. Tonkonogova. 1967. K morfologicheskoi kharakteristike ateroskleroza (po sektsionnomu materialu bol'nits Alma-Aty za 1959–1963 gg) (The morphological characteristic of atherosclerosis as indicated by autopsy materials at Alma-Ata hospital, 1959–1963), in *Trudy 4-go Vsesoyuzn. S''ezda patologoanatomov.* Moscow, p. 378.

Panfilov, Yu. A., and V. M. Rusakov. 1966. Khronicheskie nespetsificheskie legochnye zabolevaniya i ateroskleroz po sektsionnym dannym (Chronic nonspecific lung diseases and atherosclerosis in some sectional material), in *25a nauch. Sessiya Kuibyshevsk. med. in-ta.* Kyibyshev, p. 257.

Parashchak, A. P., and L. A. Shvedenko. 1963. Infarkt miokarda pri tireotoksikoze (Myocardial infarction in thyrotoxicosis). *Probl. endokrinol.* 2:109.

Parrish, H. M. 1961. Epidemiology of ischemic heart disease among white males. *J. Chron. Dis.* 14:311.

Parrish, H. M., J. C. Goldner, and S. L. Sulberg. 1966. Coronary atherosclerosis and cancer in women. *Arch. Intern. Med.* 117:639.

Pavlovskii, D. P., and B. G. Korvatskii. 1963. Funktsional'noe sostoyanie svertyvayushchei, antisvertyvayushchei i fibrinoliticheskoi sistemy krovi u bol'nykh tirotoksikozom (The activity of coagulation, anticoagulation and fibrinolytic processes of the blood in patients with thyrotoxicosis). *Vrach. delo* 12:46.

Permyakov, N. K., and A. E. Podol'skii. 1964. Revmaticheskie poroki serdtsa u lits srednego i pozhilogo vozrasta (Rheumatic lesions of the heart in elderly people). *Klin. Med.* 7:40.

Petrovskii, V. I., S. A. Davydova, and L. S. Glushchenko. 1972. O vzaimootnosheniyakh ateroskleroza i revmatizma—po dannym lipidnogo obmena (The interrelation between atherosclerosis and rheumatism—data on lipid metabolism). *Kardiologiya* 4:18.

Pietschmann, H., and F. Reinhardt. 1963. Statistisch-klinische Untersuchungen. Uber den Altersdiabetes. *Wien. Klin. Wschr.* 15:257.

Plokhinskii, N. A. 1961. *Biometriya* (*Biometric*). Novosibirsk. Akad. Nauk SSSR, Sibirsk. otd., 364 p.

Pollack, O. J. 1968. Human pancreatic atherosclerosis. *Ann. N. Y. Acad. Sci.* 149:928.

Popova, N. L. 1965. Pechen' i ateroskleroz (The liver and atherosclerosis). *Zdravookhr. Tadzhikistana* 5:84.

Pronin, Yu. I. 1961. K voprosu o svyazi ozhireniya i ateroskleroza (The correlation between obesity and atherosclerosis). *Ter. Arkh.* 11:84.

Proudfit, W. L., and E. K. Shirey. 1966. Selective cine coronary arteriography. Correlation with clinical findings in 1000 patients. *Circulation* 33:901.

Randerath, E., and P. B. Diezel. 1959. *Dtsch. Arch. Klin. Med.* 205:523.

Rapoport, Ya. L. 1935. Rasprostranenie arterioskleroza v razlichnykh otdelakh sosudistoi sistemy cheloveka i ego korrelyatsiya s nekotorymi fak torami (The distribution of atherosclerosis in various parts of the vascular system in man and its correlation with certain factors). *Arkh. Pat.* 1:66.

Rasson, G., and P. Van den Straeten. 1969. Le rôle de l'hypertension artérielle dans la pathologie coronarienne. *Acta Cardiol.* 24:83.

Ratner, N. A. 1971. *Bolezni pochek i gipertoniya* (Diseases of the kidneys and hypertension). Meditsina, Moscow.

Rau, H. 1956. Zur Bedeutung der Chronischen Blutdruckerhohung für die Entstehung der Arteriosklerose. *Klin. Wschr.* 5/6:167.

Reiner, L., F. A. Jimenez, and F. V. Rodriguez. 1963. Atherosclerosis in the mesenteric circulation. *Am. Heart J.* 66:200.

Restrepo, C., M. R. Montenegro, and L. A. Solberg. 1968. Atherosclerosis in persons with selected diseases. *Lab. Invest.* 18:552.

Rivin, A. U., and S. P. Dimitroff. 1954. The incidence and severity of atherosclerosis in estrogen-treated males and in females with a hypoestrogenic or a hyperestrogenic state. *Circulation* 9:533.

Roberts, J. C., C. Moses, and R. H. Wilkins. 1959. Autopsy studies in atherosclerosis. *Circulation* 20:511.

Robertson, W. B. 1962. Some factors influencing the development of atherosclerosis. *J. Atheroscler. Res.* 2:79.

Robertson, W. B., and J. P. Strong. 1968. Atherosclerosis in persons with hypertension and diabetes mellitus. *Lab. Invest.* 13:538.

Rogers, J. H. 1957. Tuberculosis and coronary thrombosis. *Ann. Intern. Med.* 47:78.

Roguski, J., J. Durkalec, F. Hasik, F. Jaroszewski, W. Krasnik, J. Nowaczyk, J. Rachlawicz, J. Roguska, and M. Ruszkowska. 1964. Incidence of clinical criteria of atherosclerosis in hypo- and hyperthyroidism, polycythemia vera and chronic cor pulmonale (Para- and anti-atherosclerosis syndrome). *Cor et vasa* (Praha) 6:219.

Romanenko, V. D. 1965. Rol' pechinky u vydilenyi kal'tsiyu z organizmu (Role of the liver in the excretion of calcium from the body). *Fiziol. zh.* 1:88.

Root, H. F., and P. White. 1956. *Diabetes mellitus.* New York.

Rosenman, R. H., M. Friedman, and O. Byers. 1952. Observations concerning metabolism of cholesterol in hypo- and hyperthyroid rats. *Circulation* 5:589.

Rosental, S. R. 1934. Studies in atherosclerosis. *Arch. Path.* 18:473.

Royer, P., and H. Mathieu. 1962. Métabolisme du calcium dans l'insuffisance thyroidienne humaine et expérimentale. *Sem. Hop. Paris* 10:1035.

Ryvkin, I. A. 1965. Zabolevaemost' i letal'nost' ot infarkta miokarda (Morbidity and mortality from myocardial infarction). *Kardiologiya* 4:42.

Sachsse, B. 1957. Zur Frage des Herzinfarktes bei Diabetes mellitus. *Artztl. Wschr.* 12:206.

Sacks, M. J. 1960. Aortic and coronary atherosclerosis in the three racial groups in Capetown. *Circulation* 22:96.

Saefer, K. E., M. Harson, and H. Neimoeller. 1961. Effect of prolonged exposure to 15% CO_2 on calcium and phosphorus metabolism. *Proc. Soc. Exp. Biol. N.Y.* 107:355.

Samad, I. A., and T. N. Noehren. 1965. Myocardial infarction in pulmonary emphysema. *Dis. Chest* 47:26.

Schettler, G. 1955. Rheumatismus und Arteriosklerosis. *Artzl. Wschr.* 10:604.

Schneider, E. 1936. Arteriosklerose und maligne Tumoren. *Med. Klin.* 32:1565.

Schubert, R., H. Peters, and H. Deuter. 1956. Gerontogische Besonderheiten des Diabetes mellitus. *Z. Alternsforschr.* 10:101.

Schwartz, C. J., N. S. Stenhouse, A. E. Taylor, and T. A. White. 1965. Coronary disease; severity at necropsy. *Brit. Heart J.* 27:731.

Sedov, K. R. 1966. Materialy po epidemiologii i patologii koronarnogo ateroskleroza v Irkutskoi oblasti (The epidemiology and pathology of coronary atherosclerosis in Irkutsk district). D.Sc. thesis, Moscow, Irkutsk.

Sedov, K. R. 1966. O vliyanii kharaktera trudovoi deyatel'nosti na razvitie koronarnogo ateroskleroza (The effect of the nature of physical activity on the development of coronary atherosclerosis), in *Gipertonicheskaya bolezn', koronarnyi ateroskleroz*, Irkutsk, p. 165.

Sedov, K. R. 1967. O chastote vtorichnogo kal'tsinoza venechnykh sosudov serdtsa i aorty (The frequency of secondary calcification of coronary vessels and the aorta), in *Trudy 4-go vsesoyuzn. S''ezda patologoanatomov*, Moscow, p. 354.

Sementsov, P. N. 1962. Ateroskleroticheskoe porazhenie sosudov pri rake (Atherosclerotic lesions of the vessels in carcinoma). *Arkh. Pat.* 7:49.

Shalevich, M. A., and G. E. Sarankin. 1962. O razvitii ateroskleroza u bol'nykh khronicheskimi nespetsificheskimi zabolevaniyami legkikh (The development of atherosclerosis in patients with chronic lung diseases). *Ter. Arkh.* 9:38.

Shamarin, P. I. 1968. O sochetanii revmaticheskikh porokov serdtsa s ateroskleroticheskim protsessom (The combination of rheumatic cardiac lesions with the atherosclerotic process). *Kardiologiya* 1:66.

Shapiro, Ya. E. 1966. Ob ateroskleroze arterii bol'shogo kruga pri diffuznom pnevmoskleroze s emfizemoi i khronicheskim legochnom serdtse (Atherosclerosis of the arteries of the systemic circulation in diffuse pneumosclerosis with emphysema and chronic cor pulmonale). *Ter. Arkh.* 3:16.

Sharlai, R. I. 1958. Rol' funktsii shchitovidnoi zhelezy v razvitii ateroskleroza (The role of the thyroid in the development of atherosclerosis). *Vrach. delo* 11:1131.

Shigeo-Okinaka. 1963. Epidemiological and pathological aspects of coronary artery disease in Japan. *Ann. N.Y. Acad. Sci.* 97:920.

Shkhvatsabaya, I. K. 1964. Znachenie nervnogo faktora v patogeneze infarkta miokarda (The significance of the neural factor in the pathogenesis of myocardial infarction). *Ter. Arkh.* 7:126.

Shkhvatsabaya, I. K., and V. I. Metelitsa. 1971. Epidemiologicheskii podkhod v izuchenii ateroskleroza, ishemicheskoi bolezni serdtsa i arterial'noi gipertonii (The epidemiological approach to the study of atherosclerosis, ischemic heart disease, and arterial hypertension). *Kardiologiya* 2:5.

Shmelev, N. A. 1957. Gormony kory nadpochechnikov i ikh primenenie pri tuberkuleze (The hormones of the adrenal cortex and their application in tuberculosis). *Probl. Tub.* 3:20.

Shulz, M., and F. Klinge. 1933. Das Gewebsbild des Fieberhaften Rheumatismus. 13. Mitteilung. Aortitis rheumatica und Arteriosclerose. *Virchows Arch. Path. Anat.* 288:717.

Shvarts, I. S. 1967. *Sakharnyi diabet i ateroskleroz* (Diabetes mellitus and atherosclerosis). Privolzh. Kn. Izd., Saratov, 68 p.

Simagina, V. A., E. Ya. Petrushev, L. I. Shchevel, L. I. Elmanova, B. V. Veselov, M. Ya. Levin, and N. I. Tarova. 1968. K voprosu o koronarnom ateroskleroze pri khronicheskikh nespetsificheskikh zabolevaniyakh legkikh (Coronary atherosclerosis in chronic lung diseases). *Kardiologiya* 2:65.

Simborg, D. W. 1970. The status of risk factors and coronary heart disease. *J. Chron. Dis.* 22:515.

Sinapins, D. 1964. Zur Morphologie der Fettresorbtion bei Atherosklerosis der Coronararterien. *Virchows Arch. Path. Anat.* 338:1500.

Siperstein, M. 1964. Rasstroistva zhirovogo obmena pri diabeta (Disorders of lipid metabolism in diabetes), in *Diabetes* (R. Williams, ed.). Translated from English. Meditsina, Moscow, p. 90.

Sipovskii, P. V., and Z. A. Vlasova. 1961. Zabolevanie aterosklerozom po sektsionnym dannym Leningrada za 1954–1958 gg (Atherosclerosis as per necropsy data in Leningrad, 1954–1958). *Klin. Med.* 5:65.

Skvortsov, M. A. 1938. Gistomorfologiya revmaticheskogo miokardita i ee klinicheskoe znachenie (Histology of rheumatic myocarditis and its clinical significance). *Arkh. Pat.* 2:7.

Smolenskii, V. S. 1960a. O metodakh otsenki stepeni eksperimental'nogo ateroskleroza (The methods of assessing the degree of experimental atherosclerosis). *Byull. Eksper. Biol.* 6:111.

Smolenskii, V. S. 1960b. Ov ateroskleroze arterii bol'shogo kruga krovoovrashcheniya u bol'nykh khronicheskim netuberkuleznym zabolevaniem legkikh (Atherosclerosis of the arteries of the systemic circulation in patients with chronic non-tuberculous diseases of the lungs). *Ter. Arkh.* 4:38.

Smolenskii, V. S. 1964. *Bolezni aorty* (*Diseases of the aorta*). Meditsina, Moscow, 283 p.

Smol'yannikov, A. V. 1970. Patologoanatomicheskii diagnoz i epikriz na sovremennom etape (Pathological diagnosis and the epicrisis of today). *Arkh. Pat.* 8:49.

Smol'yannikov, A. V., and T. A. Naddachina. 1967. O patogeneticheskikh osobennostyakh infarkta miokarda na razlichnykh etapakh koronarnoi nedostatochnosti (The pathological features of myocardial infarction in the various stages of coronary insufficiency), in *Trudy 4-go Vsesoyuzn. S''ezda patologoanatomov*., Moscow, p. 112.

Spain, D. M., D. J. Nathan, and M. Gellis. 1963. Weight, body type, and prevalence of coronary atherosclerotic heart disease in males. *Am. J. Med. Sci.* 245:97.

Spasskaya, M. G. 1967. Khronicheskaya rasslaivayushchaya anevrizma na pochve revmaticheskogo aortita (Chronic dissecting aneurysm in rheumatic aortitis). *Arkh. Pat.* 7:68.

Spektor, A. M. 1967. Revmatizm i ateroskleroz (Rheumatism and atherosclerosis). *Kazansk. med. zh.* 4:79.

Stamler, J. 1962. Interrelationships between two diseases—hypertension and atherosclerosis. *Am. J. Cardiol.* 9:743.

Stamler, J. 1971. Myocardial infarction—progress in primary prevention. *Brit. Heart J.* 33(Suppl.):145.

Stamler, J., D. Berkson, and H. A. Lindberg. 1972. Risk factors, in *The Pathogenesis of Atherosclerosis* (R. W. Wissler and J. C. Geer, eds.), Baltimore, p. 41.

Steiner, A., and B. Domanski. 1942. Serum cholesterol and atherosclerosis in chronic glomerulonephritis. *Am. J. Med. Sci.* 204:79.

Stepanov, S. A. 1966. Gistologicheskie i gistokhimicheskie izmeneniya ostrovkov podzheludochnoi zhelezy pri ateroskleroz i gipertonicheskoi bolezni (Histological and histochemical changes in the Islets of Langerhans in atherosclerosis and hypertension). *Probl. endokrinol.* 6:109.

Sternby, N. H. 1968. Atherosclerosis in a defined population. *Acta Path. Microbiol. Scand.* 194(Suppl.):216.

Sternby, N., R. Vanecek, A. Vikhert, A. Kagan, and K. Uemura. 1965. Correlation of the type and extent of atherosclerosis in the aorta and coronary arteries studied at autopsy. *Bull. WHO* 33:741.

Straus, R., M. Wurm, W. E. Myers, and D. Salkin. 1962. Distribution of serum lipids in tuberculous patients and their relation to clinical coronary heart disease. *Am. J. Clin. Path.* 37:339.

Strong, J. P., and H. C. McGill, Jr. 1969. The pediatric aspects of atherosclerosis. *J. Atheroscler. Res.* 9:251.

Strukov, A. I. 1961. Dinamika tkanevykh izmenenii pri revmatizme (The dynamics of tissue changes in rheumatic disease). *Arkh. pat.* 7:3.

Strukov, A. I., and A. G. Beglyaryan. 1963. *Patologicheskaya anatomiya i patogenez kollagenovykh boleznei* (*Pathological picture and pathogenesis of collagen diseases*). Medgiz, Moscow, 323 p.

Stupina, A. S. 1950. Patomorfologicheskie izmeneniya v okoloshchitovidnykh zhelezakh pri razlichnykh zabolevaniyakh (Pathological changes in the parathyroid glands in various diseases). Abstract of Ph.D. thesis, Kharkov.

Sumarokov, A. V., and A. A. Fokina. 1967. Osobennosti kliniki i simptomatologii revmaticheskikh porokov serdtsa pri ateroskleroze (The clinical features and symptoms of rheumatic heart disease in atherosclerosis). *Sov. Med.* 7:92.

Syurin, A. A. 1966. Svertyvaemost' krovi i protrombirovanie pri serdechno-sosudistoi nedostatochnosti (The clotting time and prothrombin time in cardiovascular failure). Abstract of D.Sc. thesis, Moscow.

Tagi-Zade, Z. A. 1967. Ateroskleroz i svertyvanie krovi pri razlichnykh funktsional'nykh sostoyaniyakh shchitovidnoi zhelezy (Atherosclerosis and coagulation in various disorders of the thyroid gland). Abstract of D.Sc. thesis, Baku.

Talalaev, V. T. 1929. *Ostryi revmatizm* (Acute rheumatism). Gos. Med. Izd., Moscow, 228 p.

Tatarskii, V. V., and V. D. Tsinzerling. 1950. O vliyanii tireoidina na obratnoe razvitie eksperimental'nogo ateroskleroza u krolika (The effect of thyroxine on the reversal of experimental atherosclerosis in rabbits). *Arkh. pat.* 1:88.

Tejada, C., J. Strong, and H. MacGill. 1958. *Arkh. pat.* 9:22.

Texon, M., A. M. Imparato, and M. Helpern. 1965. The role of vascular dynamics in the development of atherosclerosis. *JAMA* 194:1226.

Thomas, W. A., K. T. Lae, and E. R. Rabin. 1956. Fatal acute myocardial infarction in diabetic patients. *Arch. Intern. Med.* 98:489.

Tichy, J., H. Svabovc-Tiche, and V. Maly. 1953. *Cas. Les Ces.* 92:1005.

Tiedemann, R. 1957. Arteriosklerosis bei Krebsleiden. *Arztl. Wschr.* 12:422.

Tiraspol'skaya, M. M., and I. M. Kostyukovskii. 1965. Ateroskleroz pri zlokachestvennykh opukholyakh (Atherosclerosis in malignant tumors), in *Teksty dokl. 2-i Khar'kovsk. mezhoblast. nauchno-prakt. konferentsii po voprosom onkologii*, Kharkov, p. 88.

Tomas, A. J. 1958. Coronary heart disease in the presence of pulmonary disease. *Brit. Heart J.* 20:83.

Tsukershtein, E. I. 1947. *Sakharnyi diabet* (Diabetes mellitus). Gos. in-t usoversh. vrachei im. S. M. Kirova, Leningrad, 337 p.

Tsyukhno, Z. I. 1964. Techenie serdechnososudistykh zabolevanii pri sakharnom diabete (The course of cardiovascular diseases in diabetes mellitus), in *Trudy Ukrainsk. in-ta eksperimental'noi endokrinologii*, 19:67.

Uemura, K., N. Sternby, R. Vanecek, A. M. Vikhert, and A. Kagan. 1964. The grading of atherosclerosis in the aorta and coronary arteries as studied at autopsy. *Bull. WHO* 31:297.

Uotila, U., E. Levonen, and J. Raekallio. 1961. On the effect of atherosclerosis and goiter on aortic histopathology and mucopolysaccharide content. *Acta Endocrinol.* 36:1.

Uspenskii, V. I., and Chzhou-Su. 1963. K kharakteristike nekotorykh storon zhirovogo obmena pri gipoksicheskoi gipoksii (The characteristic of some aspects of lipid metabolism in hypoxia). *Pat. Fiziol.* 4:60.

Vadachkoriya, G. A. 1964. *Strukturnye izmeneniya nekotorykh endokrinnykh zhelez pri eksperimental'nom ateroskleroze* (Structural changes in some endocrine glands in experimental atherosclerosis). Tbilisi, Sabchota Sakartvelo, 144 p.

Vail, S. S. 1966. Discussion on the lecture by B. I. Il'inskii and B. S. Nalimov on "The prevalence of atherosclerosis in tuberculosis." *Trudy Leningradsk. nauchn. o-va patologoanatomov*, Series 7, p. 26.

Vanecek, R., A. M. Vikhert, A. Kagan, K. Uemura, and N. Sternby. 1967. Ateroskleroz koronarnykh arterii v nekotorykh evropeiskikh gorodakh (Atherosclerosis of the coronary arteries in several European cities), in *Trudy 4-go Vsesoyuzn. S''ezda patologoanatomov*. Moscow, p. 338.

Van Liere, E. J., and J. C. Stickney. 1967. *Gipoksiya* (*Hypoxia*). Translated from English. Meditsina, Moscow, 368 p.

Vengerko, Ya. 1958. Nekotorye dannye ob ateroskleroze v sochetanii s sakharnym diabetom (Some data on atherosclerosis in combination with diabetes mellitus), in *Trudy 14-go Vsesoyuzn. S''ezda Terapevtov.*, Moscow, p. 594.

Vikhert, A. M. 1973. Ateroskleroz venechnykh arterii i koronarnaya bolezn' serdtsa (Atherosclerosis of the coronary arteries and coronary heart disease). *Ter. Arkh.* 12:107.

Vikhert, A. M., and E. F. Matova. 1967. Smert' ot ostroi koronarnoi nedostatochnosti i infarkta miokarda v pozhilom vozraste (Death from acute coronary insufficiency and myocardial infarction in elderly subjects), in *Ateroskleroz i koronarnaya nedostatochnost*. Tbilisi, p. 459.

Vikhert, A. M., and V. S. Zhdanov. 1970. O ritmicheskikh strukturakh intimy aorty (The histology of the intima of the aorta). *Arkh. Pat.* 7:68.

Vikhert, A. M., V. S. Zhdanov, and E. E. Matova. 1965. Nekotorye voprosy izucheniya epidemiologii i patologii ateroskleroza po sektsionnym materialam (Some problems in studying the epidemiology and pathology of atherosclerosis in autopsy material), in *Voprosy morfologii nekotorykh zabolevanii v Uzbekistane*, Tashkent, p. 40.

Vikhert, A. M., V. S. Zhdanov, E. E. Matova, and V. V. Alpatov. 1966. Sravnitel'naya kharakteristika ateroskleroticheskikh porazhenii aorty na okrashennykh i neokrashennykh sudanom IV preparatakh (Comparative characteristics of atherosclerotic lesions of the aorta in preparations stained with Sudan IV and in unstained preparations). *Arkh. Pat.* 8:31.

Vikhert, A. M., V. S. Zhdanov, and E. E. Matova. 1967a. Ateroskleroz aorty i venechnykh sosudov serdtsa v razlichnykh zabolevaniyakh (Atherosclerosis of the aorta and coronary arteries in various diseases). *Vestn. AMN SSSR* 4:49.

Vikhert, A. M., V. S. Zhdanov, E. E. Matova, and V. S. Yagodovskii. 1967b. Kharakterisktika vozrastnoi dinamiki ateroskleroza aorty i venechnykh arterii serdtsa po sektsionnym materialam razlichnykh gorodov (Characteristics of the age-dynamics of atherosclerosis in the aorta and coronary arteries in autopsy material from different cities), in *Vsesoyuzn. S''ezda patologoanatomov*, Moscow, p. 334.

Vikhert, A. M., K. R. Sedov, and R. I. Sokolova. 1970. *Kal'tsinoz arterii i koronarnykh sosudov* (*Calcification of the arteries and coronary vessels*). Meditsina, Moscow, 152 p.

Vilkovskii, A. L., and Yu. L. Zakhar'in. 1959. K voprosu ob uchastii legkikh v obmene veshchestv (Participation of the lungs in metabolism). *Ter. Arkh.* 6:46.

Voinova, M. Kh. 1967. Lipoliticheskaya aktivnost legkikh i pecheni pri nagruzkakh zhirom (Lipolytic activity of the lungs and liver with a lipid load). *Byull. eksper. biol.* 2:47.

Volkova, K. G. 1946. Ob ateroskleroze aorty pri alimentarnoi distrofii (Atherosclerosis of the aorta in alimentary dystrophy), in *Trudy Leningradsk. fil. Vsesoyuzn. in-ta eksperimental'noi meditsiny*, Leningrad, p. 105.

Voronkov, A. G. 1967. K kharakteristike ateroskleroza pri revmatizme (The characteristics of atherosclerosis in rheumatic disease), in *Trudy Ryazansk. med. in-ta*, 28:154.

Wang and Hu. 1957. Stepen' i chastota ateroskleroza u kitaitsev i evropeitsev (The degree and prevalence of atherosclerosis in Chinese and Europeans). *Usloviya zhizni i zdorov'e* 3:1969.

Wanscher, O., J. Clemessen, and A. Nielsen. 1951. Negative correlation between atherosclerosis and carcinoma. *Brit. J. Cancer* 5:172.

Wartman, W. B., and H. K. Hellerstein. 1948. The incidence of heart disease in 2000 consecutive autopsies. *Ann. Intern. Med.* 28:41.

Weicksel, P. 1960. Uber das Seltene Zusammentrefen von Tuberkulose und Atherosklerose. *Beitr. Klin. Tuberk.* 122:123.

Welch, C. C., L. Proudfit, F. M. Sones, E. K. Shirey, C. Sheldon, and M. Razavi. 1970. Cinecoronary arteriography in young men. *Circulation* 42:647.

Welsch, R. A., J. P. Strong, and H. G. McGill, Jr. 1961. Colloid goiter and atherosclerosis. *Circulation* 24:777.

White, M. K., J. E. Edwards, and T. J. Dry. 1950. The relationship of the degree of coronary atherosclerosis with age in men. *Circulation* 1:645.

White, P., and E. Waskow. 1948. Clinical pathology of diabetes in young patients. *South. Med. J.* 41:561.

Wilens, S. 1947. The resorption of arterial atheromatous deposits in wasting disease. *Am. J. Path.* 23:793.

Winkelstein, W., R. Lilienfeld, Jr., J. W. Pactren, and A. M. Lilienfeld. 1959. The relationship between aortic atherosclerosis and cancer. *Brit. J. Cancer* 13:606.

Wuest, J. H. Jr., T. J. Dry, and J. E. Edwards. 1953. The degree of coronary atherosclerosis in bilaterally oophorectomized women. *Circulation* 7:801.

Yagudaev, A. M. 1968. Morphogenez ateroskleroza aorty pri razlichnykh formakh endemicheskogo zoba u naseleniya Ferganskoi doliny (Morphogenesis of atherosclerosis of the aorta in various types of endemic goiter in the people of Fergan Valley). Abstract of Ph.D. thesis, Moscow.

Yudanova, I. S., and M. N. Solodun. 1964. Inkretornaya funktsiya podzheludochnoi zhelezy u bol'nykh aterosklerozom (The endocrine function of the pancreatic gland in patients with atherosclerosis). *Ter. Arkh.* 11:50.

Yushina, G. I. 1967. Nekotorye pokazateli svertyvayushchei i fibrinoliticheskoi sistem krovi u bol'nykh emfizemoi legkikh (Some coagulation and fibrinolytic properties of the blood in patients with emphysema). *Ter. Arkh.* 1:24.

Yusupov, I. 1971. Morfogenez ateroskleroza venechnykh arterii serdtsa pri razlichnykh formakh endemicheskogo zoba u naseleniya Ferganskoi doliny (Morphogenesis of atherosclerosis of the coronary arteries in various types of endemic goiter in the population of Fergan Valley). Ph.D. thesis, Moscow and Andizhan.

Zaitsev, V. F., and V. G. Ananchenko. 1967. Znachenie tromboobrazovaniya v patogeneze ateroskleroza (The importance of thrombus formation in the pathogenesis of atherosclerosis). *Kardiologiya* 1:83.

Zhdanov, V. S. 1966. Ob ateroskleroze pri tsirrozakh pecheni (Atherosclerosis in cirrhosis of the liver), in *Gipertonicheskaya bolezn, koronarnyi ateroskleroz*. Irkutskii gos. med. in-ta., Irkutsk, 96 p.

Zhdanov, V. S. 1969. O vliyanii nekotorykh zabolevanii na razvitie ateroskleroticheskikh izmenenii v aorte i koronarnykh arteriyakh serdtsa (The effect of various diseases on the development of atherosclerotic changes in the aorta and coronary arteries). D.Sc. thesis, Moscow.

Zhdanov, V. S., A. M. Vikhert, and G. E. Sarankin. 1973. Ob obratnom razvitii ateroskleroza u cheloveka (Reversal of atherosclerosis in man). *Kardiologiya* 2:39.

Zhukov, N. A. 1959. K voprosu o razvitii sakharnogo diabeta pri gipertonicheskoi bolezni (The development of diabetes mellitus in hypertension). *Sov. Med.* 8:59.

Zhukov, N. A. 1964. O roli vozrastnykh izmenenii insulyarnogo apparata podzheludochnoi zhelezy v razvitii sakharnogo diabeta u lits pozhilogo vozrasta (Role of age changes in the

Islets of Langerhans of the pancreas in the development of diabetes mellitus in elderly subjects). *Sov. Med.* 9:13.

Zschoch, H. 1964. Häufigkeit und Korrelation der Leberzirrhose in Sektionsgut. *Z. Ges. Inn. Med.* 19:162.

Zschoch, H. 1967. *Trudy 4-go Vsesoyuznogo S"ezda patologoanatomov*. Moscow, p. 341.

Subject Index